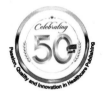

Step by Step®
ULTRASOUND IN OBSTETRICS

Third Edition

Editor-in-Chief

Narendra Malhotra
MD FICMCH FICOG FRCOG FICS FMAS FIAP
President, INSARG, Past President, FOGSI/IFUMB/ISPAT/ISAR
Vice President, WAPM/SAFOG
Managing Director, Global Rainbow Health Care & MNMH(P) Ltd
Agra, Uttar Pradesh, India
Professor, Sarajevo School of Science and Technology, Croatia

Associate Editors

Nidhi Gupta MS FICMCH FICOG
Past President, Agra Obstetrical & Gynecological Society
Professor, Department of Obstetrics and Gynecology
SN Medical College, Agra, Uttar Pradesh, India

Neharika Malhotra
MD (Gold Medalist) DRM (Germany) FICMCH
Fellow ICOG (Rep Med) ICOG (USG)
Joint Secretary, FOGSI, Chair YTP Committee, FOGSI
Director and Consultant, Global Rainbow IVF & MNMH(P) Ltd
Agra, Uttar Pradesh, India

Jaideep Malhotra
MD FICMCH FICOG FRCOG FRCPI FMAS
President, SAFOM/ISPAT
Past President, IMS/ISAR/FOGSI/ASPIRE
Managing Director, ART—Global Rainbow IVF & MNMH(P) Ltd
Agra, Uttar Pradesh, India

Kuldeep Singh MBBS FAUI FICMCH
Consultant Ultrasonologist
Dr Kuldeep's Ultrasound and Color Doppler Clinic
New Delhi, India

JAYPEE BROTHERS MEDICAL PUBLISHERS
The Health Sciences Publisher
New Delhi | London

Jaypee Brothers Medical Publishers (P) Ltd

Headquarters
Jaypee Brothers Medical Publishers (P) Ltd
EMCA House, 23/23-B
Ansari Road, Daryaganj
New Delhi 110 002, India
Landline: +91-11-23272143, +91-11-23272703
+91-11-23282021, +91-11-23245672
Email: jaypee@jaypeebrothers.com

Corporate Office
Jaypee Brothers Medical Publishers (P) Ltd
4838/24, Ansari Road, Daryaganj
New Delhi 110 002, India
Phone: +91-11-43574357
Fax: +91-11-43574314
Email: jaypee@jaypeebrothers.com

Overseas Office
J.P. Medical Ltd
83 Victoria Street, London
SW1H 0HW (UK)
Phone: +44 20 3170 8910
Fax: +44 (0)20 3008 6180
Email: info@jpmedpub.com

Website: www.jaypeebrothers.com
Website: www.jaypeedigital.com

© 2021, Jaypee Brothers Medical Publishers

Inquiries for bulk sales may be solicited at: jaypee@jaypeebrothers.com

Step by Step® Ultrasound in Obstetrics

First Edition: 2004

Second Edition: 2008

Third Edition: **2021**

ISBN: 978-93-5270-904-5

Printed at: Samrat Offset Pvt. Ltd.

Dedicated to

All the ultrasound lovers

Preface to the Third Edition

"Use sound to see better
Turn on the color to improve your image
Shift to the 3rd and 4th dimension
Heal with sound"

Ultrasonography has become a very important diagnostic tool in obstetrics and is now used extensively to determine anatomic parameters, such as location of the placenta, fetal presentation and lie and biometric measurements of the fetus to date the gestation.

It is also used to assess fetal growth and to diagnose congenital anomalies. In fact, the indications of ultrasound in obstetrics have become so numerous, information obtained so valuable that, ultrasonography equipment has moved from the radiology department to the labor room and obstetrician's office.

After a great enthusiasm shown to our earlier editions, by all the readers we have come out with a new edition adding chapters—basics in ultrasonography, training and syllabus for FOGSI-ICOG certificate courses in ultrasound medicine, a detail account of filling up form, PCPNDT Act, Ergonomics in reducing injury risk in sonography has been described in detail. The book is well illustrated with recent ultrasound images for the busy practitioners as ready reference.

Almost 50 tables and flowcharts have been incorporated in the book to act as a ready reckoner for the busy obstetrician.

We hope the readers will be benefited by this book.

Narendra Malhotra
Nidhi Gupta
Neharika Malhotra
Jaideep Malhotra
Kuldeep Singh

Preface to the First Edition

Today ultrasound is the mainstay investigation in all fields of medicine. The widespread use of ultrasound has brought this wonderful technology to the consulting rooms of the practising gynecologists. It is now impossible to even conceive a modern obstetric care unit without ultrasound and it is impossible to practise infertility and gynecology without a transvaginal probe which has added the dimension of imaging with palpation.

The law in India mandates that each machine and the sonologist be licensed to practise ultrasound under the PNDT Act for which training and updating is required.

There are numerous textbooks and reference books on ultrasound but our aim to bring out this handy series of Step by Step Ultrasound in Obstetrics is to simplify the indications, steps and the interpretations of this wonderful technology.

We hope the readers will be benefited by this book.

Kuldeep Singh
Narendra Malhotra

Acknowledgments

Our heartiest thanks to our parents, elders, teachers, spouses, siblings, our sons, daughters and our friends who have helped us step by step at every step of our ambitious project of step by step series.

We were introduced to interventional sonography by Ananda Kumar (Singapore), Rajat Goswamy (UK), Asim Kurjak and Sanja Kupesic (Croatia), Prof Alfred Kratrochwil (Austria), Ashok Khurana, Ambarish Dalal, Pratap Kumar, Bhupendra Ahuja, Dr PK Shah, Jatin P Shah and Pranay Shah and many others who taught us small tricks of the trade at each step of our life.

We are indebted to Prof Struat Campbell and Prof Asim Kurjak for teaching us imaging and grateful to Ian Donald School, India and INSUOG.

Special thanks to Dr Rahul Gupta and Nitin Agarwal of Rainbow 4D imaging center for all the images.

Editor-in-Chief
Narendra Malhotra

Contents

Basics in Ultrasonography

1.1 BASIC PHYSICS

In order to obtain the best image possible, basic fundamentals of ultrasound wave physics must be understood and applied.

Audible Sound Waves

Audible sound waves lie between 20 and 20,000 Hz: Ultrasound uses sound waves between l and 30 MHz.

Sound Wave Propagation

Sound waves need a media to travel and do not exist in a vacuum, and propagation in gases is poor because the molecules are widely separated.

The closer the molecules are, the faster the sound wave moves through a medium, so bone and metals conduct sound exceedingly well.

Effect on Image

Air-filled lungs and gut containing air conduct sound so poorly that they cannot be imaged with ultrasound instruments. Structures behind them cannot be seen.

A neighboring soft-tissue or fluid-filled organ must be used as a window through which to image a structure that is obscured by air.

An acoustic gel must fill the space between the transducer and the patient, otherwise sound will not be transmitted across the air-filled gap.

Bone conducts sound at a much faster speed than soft tissue.

Because ultrasound instruments cannot accommodate the difference in speed between soft tissue and bone, current systems do not image bone or structures covered by bone.

Pulse-Echo Principle (Figs.1.1A and B)

Because the crystal in the transducer is electrically pulsed, it changes shape and vibrates, thus producing sound waves that propagates through the tissues.

The crystal emits sound for a brief moment and then waits for the returning echo reflected from the structures in the plane of the sound beam.

When the echo is received the crystal again vibrates, generating an electrical voltage comparable to the strength of the returning echo.

Effect on Image

Greyscale imaging shows echoes in varying levels of grayness, depending on the strength of the interface.

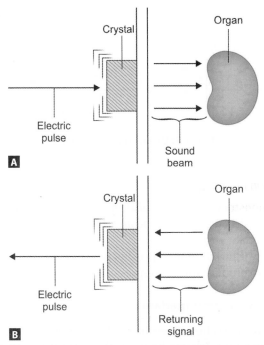

Figs. 1.1A and B: The pulse-echo principle. (A) The electrical pulse strikes the crystal and produces a sound beam, which propagates through the tissues. (B) Echoes arising from structures are reflected back to the crystal, which in turn vibrates, generating an electrical impulse comparable to the strength of the returning echo.

Beam Angle to Interface (Fig. 1.2)

The strength of the returning echo is related to the angle at which the beam strikes the acoustic interface. The more nearly perpendicular the beam is, the stronger the returning echo will be smooth. Interfaces at right angles to the beam are known as *specular reflectors.*

Echoes reflected at other angles are known as *scatter.*

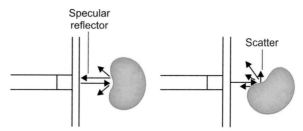

Fig. 1.2: Beam angle to interface.

Effect on Image

To demonstrate the borders of a body structure, the transducer must be placed so that the beam strikes the borders more or less at a right angle.

It is worthwhile to attempt to image a structure from different angles to produce the best representation (Fig. 1.3).

Tissue Acoustic Impedance

The returning echo's strength also depends on the differences in acoustic impedance between the various tissues in the body.

Acoustic impedance relates to tissue density; the greater the difference in density between two structures, the stronger the returning interface echoes defining the boundaries between those two structures on the ultrasound image will be.

Effect on Image

Structures of differing acoustic impedance (such as the gallbladder and the liver) are much easier to distinguish from one another than are structures of similar acoustic texture (e.g. kidney and liver).

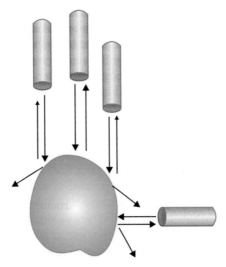

Fig. 1.3: When visualizing a structure, it is important to scan at several different angles to find the best possible interface *(thick arrows)*. Only a few echoes return from the interfaces at an oblique angle to the beam—specular reflections *(thin arrows)*. Most of the echoes are scattered.

Absorption and Scatter

Because much of the sound beam is absorbed or scattered as it travels through the body, it undergoes progressive weakening (attenuation).

Effect on Image

Increased absorption and scatter prevent one from seeing the distal portions of a structure. In obese patients, the diaphragm is often not visible beyond the partially fat filled liver.

Fibroids may absorb so much sound that their posterior borders may be difficult to define.

Transducer Frequency

Transducers come in many different frequencies—typically 2.5, 3.5, 5, 7, and 10 MHz.

Increasing the frequency improves resolution but decreases penetration.

Decreasing the frequency increases penetration but diminishes resolution.

Effect on Image

Transducers are chosen according to the structure being examined and the size of the patient. The highest possible frequency should be used because it will result in superior resolution. Pediatric patients can be examined at 5–10 MHz.

Lower frequencies (e.g. 2.5 MHz) permit greater penetration and may be needed to scan larger patients.

Beam Profile (Fig.1.4)

The sound beam varies in shape and resolution.

Close to the skin, it suffers from the effect of turbulence, and resolution here is poor. Beyond the focal zone, the beam widens.

Effect on Image

Information that appears to be present in the near field may actually be an artifact. Structures beyond the focal zone are distorted and difficult to see. A structure as small as a pinhead may appear to be half a centimeter wide.

Transducer Focal Zone

Sound beams can be focused in a similar fashion to light. Most systems use electronic focusing which permits the transducer to be focused at one or more variable depths. The sonographer can alter the focus level electronically.

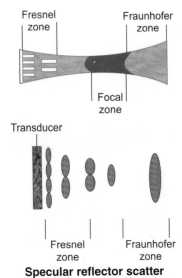

Specular reflector scatter

Fig. 1.4: Diagram of the waveforms in a sound beam. Unequal waveforms in the near field (Fresnel zone). Widening of focal beam (Fraunhofer zone) beyond the focal zone.

Effect on Image

To achieve high resolution choose a transducer with a proper focal zone or use an electronically focusing set at the right depth.

1.2 INSTRUMENTATION

Transducers

The transducer assembly consists of five main components (Fig. 1.5).

1. The *transducer crystal* is composed of a piezoelectric material, most commonly lead zirconate titanate. It converts the electrical voltage into acoustic energy upon transmission and acoustic energy to electrical energy upon reception.

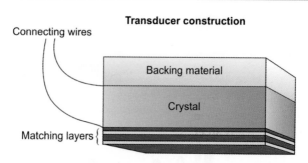

Fig. 1.5: Diagram showing transducer construction. Matching layers of material decrease the size of the main bang acoustic interface that occurs between the crystal and the skin. Backing material acts as a damping tool to stop secondary reverberations of the crystal. The crystal is constructed of piezoelectric material, which can convert electrical impulses into sound waves and vice versa.

2. The *matching layers* lie in front of the transducer element and provide an acoustic connection between the transducer element and the skin.
3. *Damping material* is attached to the back of the transducer element to decrease secondary reverberations of the crystal with returning signals.
4. The *transducer case* provides a housing for the crystal and damping layer and insulation from interference by electrical noise.
5. The *electronic cable* contains the bundle of electrical wires used to excite the transducer elements and receive the returned electrical impulses.

There are several types of transducer elements:

1. **Mechanical transducers**
   - The transducer crystal is physically moved to provide steering for the beam
   - Less commonly used in modern equipment than phased-array transducers

- Often used in volume transducers for 3D or 4D applications.

2. **Oscillating transducer (volume)**
   - The drive motor and transducer array are housed in the transducer case
   - The motor drives the transducer array back and forth to generate an image (Fig. 1.6).

3. **Electronically steered systems**
   - In this type of transducer, multiple piezoelectric elements are used and a separate electrical signal is provided for each element
   - Steering and focusing occur by sequentially exciting individual elements across the face of the transducer
   - Focusing is controlled electronically by the operator through placement of the focal zone or focus caret
   - The images are displayed in a sector, vector, linear, or curved linear format.

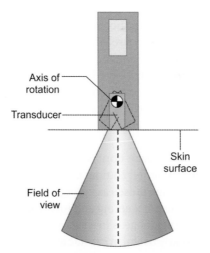

Fig. 1.6: Oscillating transducer (volume).

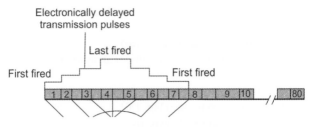

Fig. 1.7: Linear sequenced arrays.

a. ***Linear sequenced arrays***
   – Multiple transducer elements are mounted on a straight or curved bar.
   – Groups of elements are electronically pulsed at once to act as a single larger element
   – Pulsing occurs sequentially down the length of the transducer face, moving the sound beam from end to end (Fig. 1.7)
   – Linear arrays produce a rectangular shaped image which is used in breast, small parts, vascular, and musculoskeletal imaging
   – Curved arrays provide a large fan-shaped image with a curved apex. These transducers are most commonly used in obstetric, gynecologic, abdominal, and endocavity imaging.

b. ***Phased array***
   – The phased array consists of multiple transducer elements mounted compactly in a line
   – All elements are pulsed as a group with small time delays to provide beam steering and focusing
   – The resulting image is in a sector or vector format and is particularly useful in cardiac and intercostal imaging (Fig.1.8).

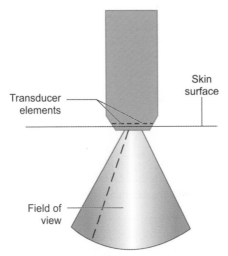

Fig. 1.8: Wedged-shaped field.

Matrix Array (Multi-O Array, 1.5D Array, 2D Array) Transducers:
- This type of transducer utilizes multiple rows of elements to form a matrix of crystals (Fig. 1.9)
- Through the use of multiple pulses, these crystals may be pulsed in sequence to create a very thin elevation plane (slice thickness), which yields increased resolution.

Hanafy Lens Technology

- This is another technique used to create a very thin slice thickness that is uniform throughout the field of view
- With this technology, the transducer crystals are cut in a planoconcave fashion (Figs. 1.10 and 1.11), which creates crystals that are thin in the center and thicker at the edges

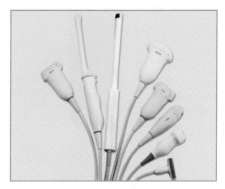

Fig. 1.9: A variety of transducers are available for specific purposes.

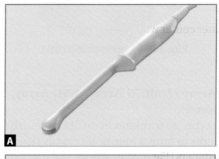

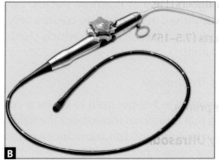

Figs. 1.10A and B: Transvaginal transducer. Transesophageal echocardiography transducer.

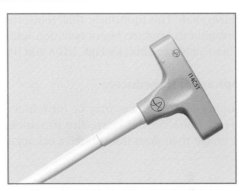

Fig. 1.11: Intraoperative transducers are designed to allow easy access to anatomy.

- The thinner center will ring at a higher frequency (focusing in the near field), and the thicker edges will ring at a lower frequency (focusing in the far field), automatically creating a uniform elevation plane (slice thickness) throughout the field of view.

Special Transducers

Special transducers (Fig. 1.11) have been produced to help view specific areas:
- Small parts (7.5–15MHz) transducer
- Rectal transducers in longitudinal (linear) and transverse (radial) configurations (biplane)
- Biopsy transducer
- Doppler probes.

Endocavity Ultrasound Systems

The transducer array, which can be a linear, curved, or phased array (or mechanical sector) scanner, is placed at the end of the transducer shaft. This transducer shaft is inserted into the rectum or vagina to produce high-resolution images of the male or female pelvic organs (*see* Figs. 1.10A and B).

Transesophageal Transducers

A transesophageal transducer may be introduced into the esophagus to visualize the heart and provides a higher resolution image than does transthoracic echocardiography (Fig. 1.12).

Intraluminal and Intracardiac Transducers

• Smaller transducers at the ends of catheters can be introduced into vessels, the biliary duct, or the ureter (transluminal transducers)

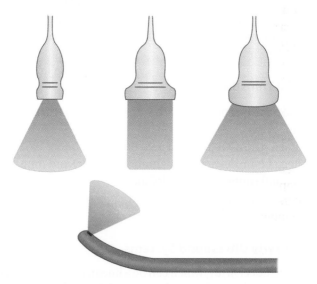

Fig. 1.12: Echocardiography transducer.

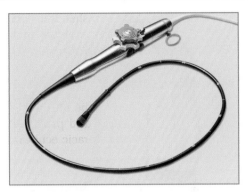

Fig. 1.13: Intraesophageal cardiac probe.

- These transducers allow close visualization of the anatomy that is being examined, but are not commonly used
- Intracardiac catheters have been developed more recently. A small catheter (IOF or *BF),* which may be introduced into the right heart (Fig. 1.13), provides very high-resolution imaging and may be used for interventional and electrophysiology applications.

Operative Systems

Standard ultrasound systems are modified so they can be used in a sterile fashion in the operating room. Special high-frequency ultrasound probes are used for this purpose (Fig. 1.14). Intraoperative transducers are designed with a size and shape to allow easy handling and positioning during intraoperative procedures.

Transducer Formats

There are a variety of transducer formats available in modern equipment, each suited to particular scanning applications.

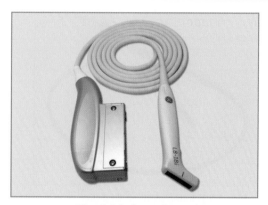

Fig. 1.14: Operative probes.

Linear array: The linear format provides a rectangular image. This transducer is most useful in "small parts" and vascular imaging.

Vector: A vector format provides a trapezoidal image. This small foot-print transducer is often used in abdominal, gynecologic, and obstetric applications.

Sector: The sector image is wedge-shaped and is commonly used in cardiac, abdominal, gynecologic, obstetric, and transcranial imaging.

Curved array: A curved array transducer will provide a large field of view with a convex near field. This transducer is most commonly used in obstetrics; however, other applications include abdominal and gynecologic imaging.

NEW TECHNIQUES FOR IMPROVING THE IMAGE

3D Imaging Systems

- 3D imaging capabilities have been increasing in popularity' over recent years

- It is most commonly used in obstetric and cardiac imaging to evaluate the surface of structures or to evaluate orthogonal planes
- It utilizes specialized transducers which relate the transducers position to the ultrasound system allowing for a very accurate display of the acoustic echoes.

4D Imaging Systems

- 4D imaging systems use specialized transducers to display the realtime motion of a 3D image
- These are most commonly used for obstetric and cardiac applications
- The transducers are commonly mechanical transducers, which are held in place while the ultrasound system controls the acquisition of the images by "rocking" the transducer crystals and displaying the 4D images.

Harmonic Imaging

- Images are obtained from returning signals, which are a multiple of the transmitted (fundamental) frequency
- The harmonic signal is created from the compression and relaxation of tissues during sound propagation
- It is helpful to reduce noise and clutter in an image, especially in technically difficult patients; however, harmonic imaging may suffer from decreased penetration due to the higher receive frequency.

Tissue Harmonic Imaging, Pulse Inversion

- With traditional ultrasound techniques, the ultrasound system transmits a pulse of a specific frequency and receives a pulse of the same frequency. This frequency is known as the *fundamental frequency*

- As this fundamental frequency travels through tissues, the tissues compress and expand with the variations in acoustic pressure, resulting in the generation of additional ultrasound frequencies, known as *harmonics*
- The harmonic frequencies are multiples of the transmitted fundamental frequency
- The challenge for the ultrasound system is to separate the clean harmonic signals from the fundamental signals. Tissue harmonic imaging removes noise from images, especially in patients who are difficult to image
- The simplest separation method is to lengthen the transmitted pulse
- Pulse inversion techniques utilize multiple pulses on transmit which vary in phase, which is maintained on transmit and receive
- The harmonic signals generated by the tissue have a different shape and phase than that of the transmitted pulse
- By summing the received pulses, the ultrasound system cancels the fundamental frequencies (destructive interference) and adds the harmonic signals (constructive interference)
- This technique often results in reduction in frame rate.

Image Compounding

Multiple ultrasound frames are averaged together to produce an image with increased contrast resolution.

Compound Imaging/Sie Clear Multiview Spatial Compounding/Sona CT Cross Beam Imaging

Image compounding averages multiple ultrasound frames to produce an image with increased contrast resolution.

Image compounding may use image frames of varying frequency (transmit or frequency compounding) or by utilizing image frames from varying angles (spatial compounding). They are of the following types:

Frequency Compounding
- Frequency compounding uses multiple transmit pulses to obtain images of the same area with different frequencies
- It provides an increase in contrast resolution and penetration.

Spatial Compounding
- This technique interrogates the same area of interest from various locations
- By averaging these ultrasound frames, the speckle pattern is reduced and will provide an image with increased contrast resolution
- Spatial compounding may occur by varying the transmitted beam's location, varying the transducer position, or by varying the location of the receive beam.

Speckle Reduction Imaging
Speckle reduction imaging is processing algorithm that reduces image speckle. The resultant images appear smoother and have increased contrast resolution as compared to the image without speckle reduction.

Elastography
- Elastography is an ultrasound technique used to evaluate the relative stiffness of tissue as compared to the surrounding area
- Results may be qualitative or quantitative in nature.

Compression elastography: It is a qualitative imaging technique that utilizes manual compression to present the relative *stiffness of tissue through* a color or black/white overlay of the image. It is most commonly used in breast imaging .

Shear-Wave Elastography: It is a technique that utilizes an electronic push pulse to provide compression of tissues. The speed of the shear wave generated by the tissue compression may then be measured. It is most commonly used in the evaluation of the liver.

1.3 KNOBOLOGY

Learning to use the knobs effortlessly is an important part of the art of ultrasound imaging.

Gain

The system gain controls the degree of echo amplification or brightness of the image. Care must be taken with the use of gain. Too much overall gain can fill fluid-filled structures with artifactual echoes, whereas too little gain can negate real echo information.

Depth Gain Compensation

The depth gain compensation (DGC) attempts to compensate for acoustic loss of sound waves by absorption, scatter, and reflection and to show structures of the same acoustic strength with the same brightness, no matter what the depth is.

Dynamic Range (Dynamic Contrast/Log Compression)

The dynamic range (log compression) is the range of intensities from the largest to the smallest echo that a system can display. Changing the log compression does not affect the number of gray shades in the image; instead, it varies the display of the gray shades.

Edge Enhancement (Preprocessing)

The preprocessing control alters the edges of the image pixels to accentuate the transition between areas of different echogenicities, making the borders sharper.

Frequency Selection (MultiHertz)

Frequency selection allows the user to optimize the imaging for the best resolution or penetration. Increasing the frequency will improve resolution but sacrifice penetration.

Maps (Postprocessing)

Maps alter image aesthetics by placing more or less emphasis on specific echo intensities. Changing the map may aid the user in evaluating pathology.

Persistence

It is a frame-averaging function that allows echo information to be accumulated over a longer period of time. By increasing the persistence subtle tissue texture differences will be enhanced and by decreasing it the moving structures are evaluated more easily.

Speckle Reduction Imaging

Speckle reduction imaging (SRI) is an image processing algorithm that reduces image speckle for enhanced contrast resolution. Higher SRI settings result in images with a smoother appearance and increased contrast resolution, as compared to the image without speckle reduction.

Zoom

The zoom function allows image magnification by increasing the pixel size, although this change results in image degradation.

Write Zoom (Res)

With write zoom, a box is placed on the screen, and the area seen within the box can be expanded to fill the screen.

Transducer Selection

The transducer selection feature allows the user to activate the transducer of choice.

Calipers

Caliper markers are available to measure distances. The ellipsoid measurement is an added feature in most units. A dotted line can be created around the outline of a structure to calculate either the circumference or the area.

1.4 DOPPLER AND COLOR FLOW PRINCIPLES

Doppler physics as it relates to diagnostic ultrasonography concerns the behavior of high-frequency sound waves as they are reflected off moving fluid (usually blood) (Fig.1.15).

Doppler Effect

When a high-frequency sound beam meets a moving structure, such as blood flow in a vessel, the reflected sound returns

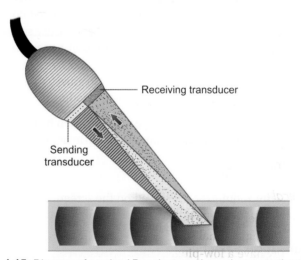

Fig. 1.15: Diagram of a pulsed Doppler transducer demonstrating the direction of the transmitted sound beam toward the flow of blood and the receiving sound beam back to the transducer.

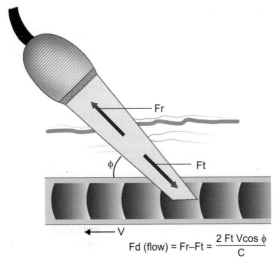

$$Fd\ (flow) = Fr-Ft = \frac{2\ Ft\ Vcos\ \phi}{C}$$

Fig. 1.16: Diagram showing the components of the Doppler equation. ϕ, angle of insonation of the vessel; C, speed of sound in tissue (–1,540 m/sec); Fr, return frequency; Ft, sending frequency; V, blood flow velocity.

at a different frequency. The speed (velocity) of the moving structure can be calculated from this frequency shift (Fig. 1.16). The returning frequency will be increased if flow is toward the sound source (transducer) and will be decreased if flow is away from the sound source.

Clinical Correlation

The Doppler effect is helpful in localizing blood vessels and determining optimal sites for velocity measurements. Veins typically have a low-pitched hum, whereas arteries have an alternating pattern with a high-pitched systolic component and a low-pitched diastolic component.

Continuous Wave Doppler

The sound beam is continuously emitted from one transducer crystal and is received by the second. Both transducers are encased in one housing.

- *Dedicated continues wave (CVV) Doppler pencil probes.*
- Imaging CW Doppler.

Clinical Correlation

Vascular surgeons use CW Doppler to check for the presence or absence of flow in superficial arteries. CW Doppler is also sometimes used to monitor umbilical artery flow. Because the cord lies in the amniotic fluid, no other confusing vessels are within the ultrasonic beam.

Pulsed Doppler

A Doppler sound beam is sent and received (pulsed) over a short period of time. Because the time that the Doppler signal takes to reach the target can be converted to distance, the depth of the site sampled is known.

The pulsed sound beam is "gated." Only those signals from a vessel at a known depth are displayed and analyzed.

Clinical Correlation

Pulsed Doppler is used to detect the presence of blood flow in a select vessel at a given depth when there are several vessels within the ultrasonic beam. Clots can appear echo-free, so a real time image may erroneously appear to show a normal vessel even if it is occluded. Doppler will detect no flow. Flow from other vessels outside the region of the gate is not analyzed because only the gated area is examined.

Flow Direction

The direction of blood flow can be discovered by assessing whether the frequency of the returning signal is above or below the baseline in a suspect vessel. Flow toward the transducer is traditionally displayed above the baseline, and flow' away from the transducer is shown below the baseline.

Clinical Correlation

Flow in the portal vein is sometimes reversed when pressure in the liver increases in portal hypertension; flow away from the liver is known as *hepatofugal* and indicates that the portal pressure is so high that flow has been reversed. A memory aid that some sonographers find useful to remember this often confusing terminology, is "fugitives flee." Flow toward the liver is known as *hepatopetal.* Flow direction analysis allows the diagnosis of the abnormal hepatofugal flow.

Flow Pattern

The pattern of flow can be assessed with Doppler ultrasound. Typically, a vein shows a continuous rhythmic flow in diastole and systole and emits a lower pitched signal than does arterial flow. Arterial flow has an alternating high-pitched systolic peak and a much lower diastolic level.

Clinical Correlation

Veins may be confused with arteries in realtime.

Flow Velocity

The velocity of blood flow can be deduced from the arterial waveform. If the peak systolic flow frequency and the angle at which the beam intersects the vessel are known, a simple formula allows the calculation of velocity (*see* Fig. 1.16). The velocity calculation formula is only accurate if the angle of the Doppler beam to the interrogated vessel is less than 60 degrees.

Clinical Correlation

Velocity is an important factor in calculating the severity of carotid stenosis. Generally, the more severe the stenosis is, the greater the velocity through the narrowed vessel will be. As the vessel becomes critically occluded, however, flow velocity will diminish.

Low-versus High-resistance Flow

Doppler flow analysis allows the detection of two types of arterial flow: a high- resistance (Fig. 1.17) and a low-resistance (Fig. 1.18) pattern.

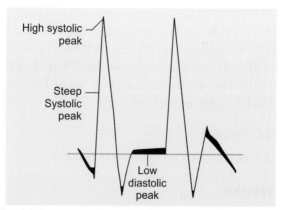

Fig. 1.17: Diagram of an arterial spectral wave form in a high resistance bed.

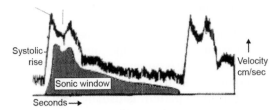

Fig. 1.18: Diagram of an arterial spectral wave form in a low resistance bed.

The high-resistance pattern has a high systolic peak and a low diastolic flow.

Low-resistance arterial systems demonstrate a biphasic systolic peak and a relatively high level of flow in diastole.

Resistance index (RI) is commonly calculated by the following formula:

$$RI = \frac{(\text{Systolic velocity Diastolic velocity})}{(\text{Systolic velocity})}$$

An alternative technique, known as the *pulsatility index* (PI), evaluates the diastolic flow in a different fashion. A cursor is run along the superior aspect of the systolic and diastolic flow envelope, and the mean is calculated by the system.

PI = (Systolic velocity – Mean flow)/(Systolic velocity)

In obstetrics, the A/B or systolic-diastolic (SID) ratio is commonly used:

$$SID = A/B = \frac{(\text{Peak systolic velocity})}{(\text{Enddiastolic velocity})}$$

All three of these parameters (RI, PI, and *SID* ratio) are just different mathematical constructs that attempt to estimate the relative difference in flow velocity between systole and diastole.

Clinical Correlation

If a high-resistance pattern is seen where there is normally a low-resistance appearance, such as in the common carotid or renal artery, vessel narrowing is present. Quantifying the severity of the resistance may help in clinical management.

A high-resistance pattern is usually seen in the vessel supplying the ovaries in the proliferative phase of the cycle.

If a low resistance pattern (RI <0.4) is seen within an ovarian mass, carcinoma is more likely.

Flow Pattern within a Vessel (Laminar Flow)

In a normal vessel, the velocity of blood is highest in the center of a vessel and is lowest closer to the wall. This condition is termed *laminar flow.* When there is a wall irregularity or if the artery is angled, the flow is distorted and may be greatest when it is closest to the vessel wall. Stenosis markedly increases the flow velocity—through an area of narrowing, whereas vessel dilatation decreases the speed of flow.

Clinical Correlation

To accurately measure the flow velocity in a tortuous carotid artery, place the sample volume (the area that is gated) at the center of the highest flow. Listening to the audible signal is useful in determining the site for optimal measurement. A high-grade stenosis will have a shrill, chirping sound.

Flow Distortion

Normal laminar flow at and immediately beyond an area of wall irregularity or stenosis is disturbed, resulting in abnormal spectral waveforms. Flow distortion (non-laminar) is characterized by high velocities in both systole and diastole. The presence of many echoes within the sonic window is termed *spectral broadening* and may indicate considerable flow disturbance.

Clinical Correlation

Flow disturbance in an artery such as the carotid may indicate pathologic atheromatous changes.

Flow Changes beyond a Narrowed Area (Poststenotic Changes)

Poststenotic changes in arterial flow may be seen in the next few centimeters beyond a narrowed area. When there is severe stenosis, the systolic peak in the poststenotic area will be lower (more rounded) with lower velocities throughout diastole. The acceleration slope of the systolic peaks (peak systole) will be diminished. This pattern is known as the *tardus et parvus* abnormality. In less severe obstruction, the spectral waveform may resume the normal high- or low-resistance flow appropriate for that artery.

Clinical Correlation

Detecting a poststenotic pattern is particularly valuable in evaluating the renal arteries because the usual site of stenosis, adjacent to the aorta, is rarely seen owing to the presence of bowel gas. Poststenotic changes may also be seen in the common carotid artery when the stenosis involves the origin of the common carotid. The waveform of the other common carotid should be evaluated for comparison. Large calcified plaques may obscure the area of stenosis, so one may be dependent on poststenotic changes to determine the severity of narrowing.

Flow Volume

The flow volume through a given vessel can be roughly estimated if the velocity of flow (using the formula shown in Figure 1.16) and the vessel diameter are known.

Clinical Correlation

The calculation of flow volume is important in situations in which a low level of flow is associated with inadequate function, e.g. penile arterial flow.

Aliasing

If there is a marked frequency shift with a high measured velocity, the signal may return after the next pulse has started. This condition is called *aliasing*.

To compensate for aliasing, increase the velocity range (PRF). Lowering the baseline may also prevent aliasing.

Clinical Correlation

If aliasing is present, the peak signal will be inaccurately measured as lower than it really is, and the severity of the stenosis will be incorrectly measured.

Color Flow Imaging

Color flow assigns different hues to the red blood cells in a vessel depending on their velocities and the direction of the blood flow relative to the transducer. This allocation is based on the Doppler principle.

Clinical Correlation

The site of maximum flow can be visualized quickly so that the pulsed Doppler gate can be inserted where the flow is highest.

Color Flow Display and Direction within a Vessel

In most systems, flow toward the transducer is allocated red, and flow away from the transducer is allocated blue. The flow velocity is displayed with faster velocities in brighter colors and slower velocities in darker colors. The fastest velocity may be displayed in yellow or white. Turbulent flow will demonstrate a mixture of colors.

As with pulsed Doppler, optimal images are only obtained at an oblique angle. If a vessel runs a straight course, flow at 90 degrees to the color box will not be displayed. The angle of the color box region of interest (ROI) can be adjusted to the left or right when linear steering is available; otherwise, the probe can be manually angled to provide the angle needed to receive the returning signals.

Clinical Correlation

Soft plaque may be missed on gray scale but a flow void will be seen using color flow. Sometimes, soft plaques may show no changes on grayscale. Once correct color allocation has been made, normal vessels will fill with color.

Knobology: Doppler and Color Flow

Range Gate Cursor (Sample Volume)

The Doppler sample volume is displayed on the B-scan image. This cursor, which may be presented as a box or two parallel bars, indicates the depth and area from which the Doppler signal is obtained.

Region of Interest

This box is used to restrict the color display of a blood flow image and to eliminate an unnecessary display of color.

Inversion and Direction of Flow and its Relation to Baseline (Doppler)

When blood flow is moving toward the transducer, sound waves of high frequency are reflected, and positive signals are seen above the baseline. Blood cells that are moving away from the transducer appear as negative signals below the baseline. Both veins and arteries can show flow in either direction because interpreting flow direction depends on the angle of the vessel to the transducer.

Color Inversion

As in spectral Doppler, the display of color is dependent on the angle of the flow to the transducer.

Color Flow Baseline

Blood flow toward the transducer will be shown within the measurable range of colors above the color bar baseline. Blood flow away from the probe will be displayed in the range of colors below the baseline.

Velocity Scale/Velocity Range/PRF (Doppler)

The range of velocities that can be seen in the spectral display is determined by the PRF value. Higher velocity vessels (e.g. carotid) requires a high PRF; therefore, the velocity range should be increased.

PRF (Color Flow)

The range of velocities used in color flow is lower compared to the spectral waveform because the average Doppler shift frequency is displayed rather than the peak velocity. Depending on the color map used, lower PRF values may present a shift to a different color, representing a slightly higher velocity flow (i.e. white or yellow).

Sweep Speed (Doppler Only)

The rate at which the spectral information is displayed can be adjusted using the sweep speed controls. A slow speed (e.g. 25 mm/sec), a moderate speed (e.g. 50 mm/sec), or a fast speed (e.g. 100 mm/sec) can be selected.

Wall Filter (Doppler)

Blood flow signals that are not wanted can be eliminated by using the wall filter.

Filter (Color Flow)

A phenomenon called *color flash,* caused by cardiac or peristaltic motion or by transducer movement, produces a flash of spurious color in an area where there is no real flow. The area of interest can be concealed by the flash artifact.

Gain (Doppler and Color Flow)

The gain controls alter the spectral waveform and the color flow image. Inadequate gain results in an image in which the vessel is incompletely filled with color or in which no spectral Doppler signal can be obtained in areas of slow flow.

Angle Correct Bar (Flow Vector)

An angle correct bar is situated within the range gate cursor. This bar should be aligned with the direction of blood flow. The angle created by the insonating ultrasound beam and this bar must be known if the flow velocity is to be deduced from the frequency of the returning Doppler signal. The angle should be less than 60 degrees.

Power Doppler

Power Doppler utilizes the amplitude of the Doppler signal to generate the ultrasound image. Areas with high concentrations of blood cells will appear in brighter colors while lower concentrations of blood cells will appear in darker colors. This technique is more sensitive for subtle flow than is conventional color flow Doppler. Power Doppler typically does not provide any directional information and is particularly useful for evaluating the presence of flow or low flow in small or subtle vessels (e.g., ovarian masses).

Audio Volume

The Doppler sound will be heard from the built-in speakers. Usually, there are independent speakers for both forward and reverse flow. The control varies the volume of the Doppler sound.

Cursor Movement Control

The cursor (range gate cursor and ROI) movement can be manipulated by means of a trackball or a joystick.

Measurements

The standard measurement unit used in displaying the spectral waveform is velocity (m/sec or cm/sec). When dealing with a high grade stenosis, obtain maximum velocities at and just beyond the area of lumen narrowing.

Pitfalls

Incorrect Angle

A waveform that appears to indicate a distal obstruction is displayed in a vessel; however, no plaque is seen in the vessel.

Correction Technique

Check the position of the ultrasound beam relation to the direction of flow. If the angle greater than 60 degrees, then the velocity is not being accurately calculated, and an abnormal waveform is created (*see* Fig. 17).

Little or No Doppler Signal in an Artery

The spectral waveform shows apparent low systolic flow and minimal diastolic flow. This may be because of:

- There may be a severe obstruction proximal to this area and in an area too difficult to evaluate with the ultrasound beam (e.g., origin of the common carotid artery)
- This patient may have diminished cardiac output

- The sample volume (gate) may not be placed where maximum flow is present
- The sample volume is too large for the small amount of flow
- The wall filters level is set too high.

Correction Technique
- Do not depend solely on the visualization of the vessel
- Color flow highlights the higher velocities in the artery and helps in gate placement, but a keen ear is more sensitive
- A higher velocity may be evident as the sound beam is angled slightly off the center of the stream
- *A larger sample size may be needed when scanning to locate the site of flow, but to obtain a more precise flow measurement within an artery, decrease the gate size*
- The wall filter *should be set at the lowest setting that does not introduce artifacts, especially when scanning a vein (a low-flow state)*

Try the following maneuvers before giving up:
- Change to another acoustic window or different incident angle
- Open up the gate setting
- Lower the velocity' range
- Use a lower frequency transducer. The patient may be too obese for a higher frequency transducer.

A High-resistance Waveform in a Low- resistance Bed

Explanation

There may be soft plaque distal to this area. If the B-scan gain is too low, soft plaque may be missed. Use color flow to outline the true patent lumen.

Aliasing

A tight stenosis causes such high velocities at the site of flow and immediately distal to the narrowed area that flow is seen above the baseline and at the lower edge of the spectral display.

When color is used, there may be peaks of color from the other end of the spectrum. A chirping sound may be heard as you angle through the stenotic area.

This may be due to the fact that, the velocity is so high that the signal wraps around itself, and peak velocities are displayed below the baseline. This problem arises because the selected PRF is too low to accurately pick up the high velocities that are occurring.

Correction Techniques

- Place the baseline at its lowest site to allow the systolic peaks to be displayed
- Increase the PRF (velocity range)
- Some units allow the B-scan image to be frozen while the Doppler signal is obtained. This will also widen the measurable velocity range
- Increase the Doppler angle, but do not exceed 60 degrees
- Decrease the insonating frequency. Most units offer a choice of several Doppler frequencies for each transducer. Otherwise, change to a lower frequency transducer
- Change to CW (not widely available on most current machines).

Inadequate Venous Signal

Venous flow is difficult to detect even when the vessel is clearly demonstrated. This may be due to:
- There may be little venous flow at rest
- The vein may be compressed by patient position
- The B-scan gain may be too low to demonstrate the clot within the vein.

Correction Technique

- Respiration affects venous flow. With inspiration and the descent of the diaphragm, pressure increases in the abdomen. Ask the patient to perform a Valsalva maneuver. As the breath is released, venous flow increases, and the venous signal will become more pronounced

- Ask the patient to flex the leg slightly and re-evaluate. Use color flow' in these instances to accentuate subtle flow
- Increase the gain and apply gentle compression to see if the vein collapses.

Audible Signal but Vessel not Seen

A venous signal can be heard, but a patent vessel cannot be visualized.

The vein may be subtotally occluded, or the presence of adjacent collaterals may cause the audible signal.

Correction Technique

Color flow will demonstrate the smaller collateral vessels as well as a small amount of residual flow in an almost occluded vessel.

Spectral Broadening

Apparent spectral broadening may be caused by too much gain or by scanning too close to the vessel wall, picking up lower velocities.

Correction Technique

Make sure the supposed spectral broadening reflects true pathology and is not just noise by comparing it to an area known to be normal.

A Flickering Image

Sometimes, it is difficult to evaluate color flow when obtaining a pulsed Doppler signal because the image flickers.

A large amount of data is being processed to generate the image for each frame of information when obtaining the Doppler signal or color flow. Therefore, the frame rate is lowered, and a flicker may occur.

Correction Technique

To reduce this flicker, evaluate one mode at a time (e.g. use color flow only) or reduce the width of the color flow box.

Color Misregistration Artifact (Color Flash)

If the transducer is rapidly moved, a flash of color related to transducer movement and not to vascular flow may develop.

Correction Technique

Use the filter to reduce noise and move the transducer slowly, using caution not to remove real vascular flow from the image.

Tissue Vibration or Transmitted Pulsation

In the region of a highly pulsatile structure such as an artery, neighboring structures may move, causing some color artifact in the surrounding tissues.

Correction Technique

Scan from a different axis if possible.

Active Peristalsis

Active peristalsis may induce a color flow artifact.

Undue Color Gain

The outline of vessels may be misregistered owing to excessive gain, so the flow appears to fill in some of the surrounding tissues (color bleed).

Correction Technique

Decrease gain so the color image corresponds to the vessel outline.

1.5 EQUIPMENT CARE AND QUALITY CONTROL

Ultrasound systems are precision instruments that require careful handling and regular maintenance to ensure optimum performance.

Preventive Maintenance

- Liquids other than contact gel should not be stored on the equipment
- The hand used to adjust control settings should be kept clean to ensure that contact gel does not affect the trackball or other functions
- Cables and transducers should be visually inspected for worn areas or cracks
- Careless placement of the transducer and cable on the machine can cause cable damage
- Transducers should be placed in proper holders to avoid stress on cables
- When taking ultrasound equipment to wards, it should be moved carefully to avoid sudden impact, which may dislodge printed circuit boards from their connectors, resulting in failure of operation
- Many ultrasound systems have cooling fans with overlying air filters to prevent deposition of dust and particles on circuit boards within the unit. These should be cleaned periodically (weekly), especially if used in carpeted areas
- Error messages should be noted and recorded for referral to service personnel.

Transducer Care

Transducers are delicate instruments and require careful handling. Transducers that have been dropped or treated roughly may have "dead" elements that no longer transmit or receive signals (due to debonding of electrodes from crystal elements).

Each time a transducer is removed from its cradle, ensure that the transducer cable is not snagged on part of the ultrasound system (such as the wheel support). The compromised length of cable may result in the transducer being pulled out of the hand as it is moved toward the patient.

Transducers should be cleaned after each patient with an alcohol sponge or transducer disinfectant, particularly if the patient has an open wound or a skin problem. Plastic freezer bags are an inexpensive means of covering the transducer to avoid contact with open wounds and to avoid contamination. Some transducers can be immersed in Cidex up to the handle for sterilization. Approximately 10 minutes of immersion is required for adequate sterilization.

Use a commercial water-soluble coupling gel to ensure good acoustic contact between the transducer and patient. Thick, high-viscosity gels are desirable when scanning the patient in an erect position because they do not slide off easily. Thicker gels are also helpful for obstetric patients with large abdomens.

Use disposable gloves when scanning a patient to avoid the risk of infection. Spread the gel around the abdomen with the transducer rather than by hand. Do not handle the controls with gel on your hand or glove.

Quality Assurance

Quality assurance tests may be tedious to perform but are worthwhile because it may be difficult or even impossible to detect calibration and measurement distortions from examination of the images alone. Clearly, major clinical problems may result if erroneous measurement data are produced. Quality assurance checks should be performed on a quarterly basis with most systems or more often if a problem a suspected e.g., if a transducer has been dropped or measurements are consistently higher or lower than expected.

Quality Control Tests

The standard tests performed to ensure that the system is working satisfactorily are:
- Aspect ratio and calibration tests
- Resolution tests (both axial and lateral)
- A comparative power output test that equates to a depth of penetration measurement.

All these tests are performed on a tissue-equivalent phantom.

Aspect Ratio and Calibration Test

The aspect ratio and calibration test measures whether distances are accurate in both directions—horizontal and vertical directions and whether these measurements are displayed accurately on a hard-copy device transducer.

Resolution

Axial and lateral resolution capability can be determined using closely spaced pins in a phantom.

Comparative Power Output

The test for comparative power output determines whether the sound beam emitted by the transducer can reach a depth adequate to see deep structures. The test is performed at full power output, and the time gain compensation is set at maximum at the area of depth visualization. The comparative power output can be calculated as follows:

$$\text{Attenuation factor } (0.7) \times \text{Depth } (7.35) \times \text{Transducer frequency } (5) = 25.725 \text{ dB}$$

This number is recorded in the quality control logbook as the output for this transducer using this phantom. Repeat tests should give the same result. For the comparison of results to be valid, all settings must be the same each time the test is undertaken. This is a useful test to see whether transmitter and/or receiver characteristics are changing over time.

Malfunction

Modem ultrasound systems are very reliable but occasionally can malfunction, resulting in disruption of images.

This is rare in modern systems, but when it occurs, it is usually obvious with clear disruption of the images.

The disruption may relate to circuitry for a specific transducer, so the equipment may still be usable with different transducers until the problem can be rectified. Occasionally, a transducer that has been selected may not initialize correctly, or its connection to the ultrasound system may be fault, but can be corrected by disconnecting and reconnecting the transducer so that it re-initializes.

Software errors occasionally occur and can often be rectified by switching the ultrasound unit off and on again, allowing the system to reboot. It may be necessary to wait 30 seconds before switching the system on again to allow time for correction of the software error.

1.6 MALPRACTICE AND ULTRASOUND

Causes of Malpractice

Legally malpractice as it relates to ultrasound comes in two forms:

1. *Battery Injury:* The patient is injured during the examination by assault or inadequate care (e.g., falls off the table). Failure to obtain informed consent is another type of "battery" injury.
2. *Negligence:* The examination is performed in a fashion that is "below the standard of care."

Standard of care is defined as the way in which a "reasonable and prudent" physician or sonographer would act under the same circumstances. In our court system, the standard of care is established in several inherent ways:

- Expert witnesses testify as to the standard of care
- Guidelines such as the American Institute of Ultrasound in Medicine (AIUM) "Practice Guidelines for the Performance of an Antepartum Obstetric Ultrasound Examination" or American Congress of Obstetricians and Gynecologists technical bulletins set national standards. There are no such laid down in our country
- Local hospital, radiology, or obstetric department policy statements also set the standard of care.

Responsibilities of the Physician or Sonographer Reporting the Study

- The physician or sonographer reporting the study is required to accurately describe the findings on the examination, including pertinent negative findings with a clinical conclusion about the presence or absence of an abnormality
- Suggestions about additional procedures or follow-up studies may be required
- Problems in the performance of the study, such as obesity or suboptimal patient position, should be covered in the narrative portion of the report
- A preliminary report is not considered legally hazardous as long as the sonographer does not attempt to make a diagnosis

- If a sonographer is working for a sonologist, the sonographer is not responsible for errors in the study, provided that the study is performed according to standards set by the sonologist, even if the study is of poor quality
- The sonographer is not liable if he or she uses a technique that creates an image that looks like pathology but is not
- Some examples of misleading findings or wrong techniques that are not the sonographers legal responsibility if uncorrected by the sonologist are the following:
  - Pseudohydronephrosis as the result of a full urinary bladder
  - Sludge-filled gallbladder due to an overgained image
  - Not following up on a pathologic finding, such as missing hydronephrosis with a pelvic mass
  - Missing a pancreatic mass by not trying different scanning techniques, such as erect scanning or having the patient drink to fill the stomach to create an acoustic window
  - Missing stones in the gallbladder or kidneys due to a failure to use a high-frequency transducer.

Although the sonographer is not held legally responsible for these errors, there is still the moral and ethical element to consider.

Responsibilities of the Physician or Sonographer Performing the Examination

- The primary responsibility is to perform a comprehensive examination that conforms to the national standards
- One should care for the patient and make sure that the patient comes to no harm by rough treatment or carelessness
- Confidentiality must be observed.

Some examples of situations in which a sonographer is liable are:

- *Physically molesting the patient*
- *Letting a patient fall, causing injury*
- *Giving the patient or accompanying doctor a wrong diagnosis*
- *Revealing confidential information about the contents of the sonogram* or disclosing any information that has adverse effects on the patient

Legally Hazardous Situations

Emergency Studies

Emergency ultrasound studies often modify clinical management from conservative to aggressive, and because any management changes hinge on the sonographic findings, the examination may be legally hazardous.

Litigation is common when a wrong diagnosis leads to immediate consequences.

Some examples of emergency situations often followed by litigation are as follows:

- *Failure to recognize ectopic pregnancy:* Few ectopic pregnancies now require immediate surgery because many are now treated with methotrexate. This has created a new risk: misdiagnosis of a normal pregnancy as an ectopic pregnancy with subsequent methotrexate treatment with survival of a deformed but viable intrauterine pregnancy
- *Failure to diagnose ovarian torsion*
- *Misdiagnosis of fetal death:* Wrongly diagnosing fetal death with the subsequent delivery of a live but damaged infant can occur
- *Failure to diagnose abruptio placenta*
- *Failure to diagnose a fetal anomaly:* Fetal abnormalities are a common cause of litigation because the monetary award for a missed anomaly is so large. Litigation related to obstetric ultrasound is many times more frequent than for all other types of ultrasound combined

- The common missed fetal abnormalities resulting in litigation are as follows:
  - Missed spina bifida
  - Hypoplastic left heart syndrome
  - Absent limb or limbs
  - Down syndrome signs
  - Hydrocephalus.

Often, the litigation concerns a basic level obstetric study in which there is a possibility of an abnormality and no recommendation is made for referral for a targeted or referral study to be performed at a specialized center.

Failure to Diagnose Major Obstetric Findings

Some obstetric ultrasound findings that have been overlooked and that have serious consequences to pregnancy management are as follows:

- *Twins or triplets:* Failure to diagnose twins or triplets can lead to severe long-term disability if the presence of twins is first discovered at delivery.
- *Unrecognized placenta previa* during a sonographic examination may lead to a major bleed at delivery.
- *Breast cancer that is misdiagnosed as merely a breast cyst:* Failure to diagnose breast cancer is the most common cause of imaging litigation. Most suits relate to mammography, but breast cancer ultrasound cases are occurring increasingly.

Substandard Reporting of the Ultrasound Study

- *Dating an obstetric study in the third trimester:* The range of possible dates for a series of obstetric measurements such as the biparietal diameter, head circumference, femur length, and abdominal circumference in the third trimester is ± three to four weeks, so accurate dating if the patient presents in the third trimester is not possible. This error is so well known that the obstetrician and radiologist share responsibility if delivery is performed before fetal viability under these circumstances

- *Dating or weight estimation with unsatisfactory measurement data:* It is not always possible to obtain a quality abdominal circumference or fetal head measurements with an unusual fetal position. Problems of this type should be noted in the report. Not reporting these problems may result in wrong clinical decisions about delivery or the presence of intrauterine growth restriction (IUGR)
- *Failure to compare the dates or weight on the current examination with earlier sonographic studies* may mean a failure to diagnose IUGR. Data from earlier sonograms should be obtained if later examinations are performed at another facility.

Tardy Reporting

- Delayed reporting of an ultrasound study or delayed transmission of an ultrasound report to the referring doctor can lead to litigation.
- Findings that change management, such as the discovery of an ectopic pregnancy or a low biophysical profile score of 0 to 2, require immediate notification to the managing physician.
- Some examples of serious consequences of a delayed report are as follows:
  - *Failure to relay a report of a placenta previa* resulted in the loss of the pregnancy in a patient with heavy vaginal bleeding
  - *Two week delay in transmitting a report of IUGR* resulting in the loss of that pregnancy.

Failure to Perform an Appropriate Ultrasound Study when a Patient Presents with a Family History of a Malformation Or a Drug History predisposing to a Malformation.

A common indication of an ultrasound study is a family history of fetal malformations or when the patient is taking drugs like valproic acid, that causes the fetal malformations. Specific views of potential malformations such as the lumbar spine with valproic acid or the face with a family history of cleft lip and palate, need to be obtained and reported.

Interventional Guidance Problems

Amniocentesis for chromosomal abnormality or to establish fetal lung maturity is still commonly performed and is standardly performed under ultrasound guidance. Suits related to fetal damage or fetal death due to the procedure still occur. Documentation of the amniocentesis site and of fetal viability after the procedure and a written report of the way in which the procedure was performed are helpful in avoiding litigation and defending complaints. By convention, only two passes are made if aspiration of amniotic fluid is unsuccessful.

MALPRACTICE INSURANCE: WHO NEEDS IT?

Any sonographer performing freelance work should invest in malpractice insurance. Sonographers employed by a hospital. or other institution do not generally need to purchase insurance because they are covered by the hospital's or clinic's policy.

Training

2.1 Theoretical Aspects
2.2 Training Parameters
2.3 Suggested Training Schedule
2.4 Prerequisite Criteria for a Trained Ultrasonologist
2.5 Mandatory Proposed Certification for the Ultrasonologist (Obstetrics and Gynecology)
2.6 Syllabus for FOGSI-ICOG Certificate Course in Ultrasound Medicine

INTRODUCTION

The practice of ultrasound and the use of diagnostic and interventional ultrasound is now a necessary tool rather than a luxury. It is impossible to even conceive an Obstetric Care Unit and Fetal Medicine Unit or even Gynecology and Infertility Diagnostic Unit without ultrasound.

To practise ultrasound in India it is mandatory to be trained in ultrasonography under proper guides and to do 100 cases minimum of Obstetrics and Gynecology. Ultrasound and 6 months of observership under a radiologist or an approved center.

2.1 THEORETICAL ASPECTS

The theoretical aspects one should know, should cover topics on physics of ultrasound, ultrasound machines and probes, how to use an ultrasound machine PNDT Act, laws of ultrasound, medicolegal aspects, methodology, patient preparations, complete obstetric ultrasound uses including use in first, second and third trimesters, diagnosis of threatened abortion, ectopic pregnancy, biometry, anomaly scanning, IUGR, placental evaluation, amniotic fluid evaluation, color Doppler uses and 3D and 4D ultrasound.

Complete gynecological ultrasound aspects include use of TVS, color and 3D in evaluating female pelvis and evaluating infertility and complete interventional procedures.

2.2 TRAINING PARAMETERS

First Level (At Least 30 Hours a Week for Two Months)

These are aimed at:
- Confirm intrauterine pregnancy
- Confirm viability
- Determine number of gestations
- Fetal biometry
- Assessment of growth
- Presentation
- Amniotic fluid assessment
- Placental assessment
- Cervix measurement
- Suspect abnormalities.

Second Level (About 100 Sessions and 300 Hours)

These are aimed at:
- Detect and specify early pregnancy problems
- Detect and specify abnormalities
- Assessment of growth restriction

- Fetal biophysical profiling
- Understanding color Doppler
- Accurately sampling various blood vessels by Doppler and analyzing them
- Knowledge of interventional procedure
- Knowledge of 3D and 4D
- Analysis of malignancies

Third Level (3 Years)

These are aimed at:
- Acquiring 3D and 4D image
- Perform interventional procedures
- Research and development
- Ability to teach basic stalls.

2.3 SUGGESTED TRAINING SCHEDULE

Viable pregnancies	10
Nonviable pregnancies	10
Normal biometry	10
Growth restrictions	10
Abnormal pregnancy (ectopic/multiple, etc.)	10
Color Doppler studies obstetrics	10
Gynecology	10
IUCDs	5
Fibroids	10
Ovarian cysts	10
Gynecological disorders	10
Transvaginal scan	10

These are minimum number of scans for Level I training.

Another 100 cases of detailed obstetric and gynecological cases for various indications including color and 3D should be logged for Level II training.

A standard reporting format for gynecology and obstetrics should be adhered to with details of different descriptive terminology.

2.4 PREREQUISITE CRITERIA FOR A TRAINED ULTRASONOLOGIST

- The ultrasonologist should be able to identify early pregnancy and emergency gynecological problems by transvaginal and transabdominal ultrasound.
    - *Early pregnancy:*
        - Fetal viability
        - Description of the gestational sac, embryo, yolk sac
        - Single and multiple gestation (chorionicity).
    - *Pathology:*
        - Early pregnancy failure
        - Ectopic pregnancy
        - Gross fetal abnormalities, such as nuchal translucency, hydropic abnormalities
        - Hydatidiform mole
        - Associated pelvic tumors.
    - *Gynecology:*
        - Normal pelvic anatomy
        - Uterine size and endometrial thickness
        - Measurement of ovaries
        - Pelvic tumors, e.g. fibroids, cysts hydrosalpinx
        - Peritoneal fluid
        - Intrauterine contraceptive devices.
- The ultrasonologist should be able to recognize the following normal fetal anatomical features from 18 weeks onwards by abdominal ultrasound.
    - *Shape of the skull:* Nuchal skinfold
    - *Brain:* Ventricles and cerebellum, choroid plexus
    - Facial profile

- – *Spine:* Both longitudinally and transversely
- – Heart rate and rhythm, size and position, four-chamber view
- – Size and morphology of the lungs
- – Shape of the thorax and abdomen
- – *Abdomen:* Diaphragm, stomach, liver and umbilical vein, kidneys, abdominal wall and umbilicus
- – *Limbs:* Femur, tibia and fibula, humerus, radius and ulna, feet and hands—these to include shape, echogenicity and movement
- – *Multiple pregnancy:* Monochorionic and dichorionic, twin-twin transfusion syndrome
- – Amount of amniotic fluid
- – Placental location
- – Cord and number of vessels.
- • *Fetal biometry:*
  - – Crown rump length, biparietal diameter, femur length, head circumference, abdominal circumference, interpretation of growth charts.
- • *Activity:* Recognize and quantify
  - – Fetal movements
  - – Breathing movements
  - – Eye movements.

2.5 MANDATORY PROPOSED CERTIFICATION FOR AN ULTRASONOLOGIST (OBSTETRICS AND GYNECOLOGY)

- • One hundred hours in 6 months, of supervised scanning to include (one year observership):
  - – Hundred gynecological examinations and early pregnancy problems (principally by transvaginal sonography but transabdominal experience also required).
  - – Two hundred obstetric scans covering the full spectrum of obstetric conditions.

- *Logbooks:* Thirty cases on one A4 page with ultrasound picture, at least 15 anomalies should be included.

These are suggested training hours and comply with the Indian Government's requirement under the modified PNDT Act.

2.6 SYLLABUS FOR FOGSI-ICOG CERTIFICATE COURSE IN ULTRASOUND MEDICINE

FOGSI-ICOG

The practice of ultrasound and the use of diagnostic and interventional ultrasound is like a stethoscope to the gynecologist today. It is impossible to even conceive an Obstetric Care unit and Fetal Medicine unit or even Gynecology and Infertility Diagnostic unit without ultrasound.

It has now been acknowledged in the modified PNDT Act that ultrasound practice can be done by a trained Gynecologist who will keep proper records as mandated by the law and will adhere to the indications, safety and ethical practice.

The Indian College of Obstetrics and Gynecology (ICOG) is the academic wing of FOGSI and the college feels the need of training its members and the members of FOGSI in the science and art of ultrasonography.

To practice ultrasound in India, it is mandatory to be trained in ultrasonography under proper guides and to do 100 cases minimum of Obstetrics and Gynecology. Ultrasound and 6 months of observership.

Keeping the above requirements in mind the ICOG along with FOGSI has devised a 6 month certificate course in Diagnostic and Interventional Obstetrics and Gynecology ultrasound for FOGSI members in India. This will be awarded to candidates who will successfully attend and complete the theoretical course and a practical training program set to a very high standard. The theoretical course is designed for both the general gynecologist and the specialized feta-maternal high-risk obstetrician. The lectures will be given by a group of experts who are leading academics in their respective fields.

Theoretical Course

The course will be held at ICOG recognized centers. The participants will be given study material (Books/Journals, etc.). A MCQ and short question evaluation test will be taken on the last day of theory lectures. The theoretical course will cover lectures on Physics of ultrasound, ultrasound machines and probes, how to use ultrasound? PNDT Act, laws of ultrasound, medicolegal aspects, methodology, patient preparations, complete obstetric ultrasound uses including use in first, second and third trimesters, diagnosis of threatened abortion, ectopic pregnancy, biometry, anomaly scanning, IUGR, placental evaluation, amniotic fluid evaluation, color Doppler uses and 3D and 4D ultrasound.

Complete gynecological uses including use of TVS, color and 3D in evaluating female pelvis and evaluating infertility. Complete Interventional procedures.

A detailed practical training will be given as observer on patients with audiovisual aids in form of CDs and videos. Hands on training will be allowed on certain patients.

Training Schedule

Aims

- Ability to visualize in two-dimensional image and a three-dimensional structure
- Hand-eye coordinations
- Supervision is essential
- Level of training depending on competence.

First Level

- Confirm intrauterine pregnancy
- Confirm viability
- Determine number of gestations
- Fetal biometry
- Assessment of growth
- Presentation
- Amniotic fluid assessment
- Placental assessment
- Cervix measurement
- Suspect abnormalities.

Second Level

- Detect and specify early pregnancy problems
- Detect and specify abnormalities
- Assessment of growth restriction
- Fetal biophysical profiling
- Understanding color Doppler
- Accurately sampling various blood vessels by Doppler and analyzing them
- Knowledge of Interventional procedure
- Knowledge of 3D and 4D
- Analysis of malignancies.

Third Level

- Acquiring 3D and 4D image
- Perform interventional procedures
- Research and development
- Ability to teach basic stalls.

Suggested Logbook for Training

Viable pregnancies	10
Nonviable pregnancies	10
Normal biometry	10
Growth restrictions	10
Abnormal pregnancy (ectopic/multiple, etc.)	10
Color Doppler studies obstetric	10
Gynecology	10
IUCSs	5
Fibroids	10
Ovarian cysts	10
Gynecological disorders	10
Transvaginal scan	10

Another 100 detailed obstetric and gynecological cases for various indications including color and 3D should be logged for Level II training.

A standard reporting format for gynecology and obstetrics should be adhered to with details of different descriptive terminology.

Organization of Ultrasound Unit

Infrastructure, documentation, quality control, computerization data storage.

Practical Training

Required Skills

- The trainee to be able to identify early pregnancy and emergency gynecological problems by transvaginal and transabdominal ultrasound.

– *Early pregnancy:*
  - Fetal viability
  - Description of the gestational sac, embryo, yolk sac
  - Single and multiple gestation (chorionicity).
– *Pathology:*
  - Early pregnancy failure
  - Ectopic pregnancy
  - Gross fetal abnormalities such as nuchal translucency, hydropic abnormalities
  - Hydatidiform mole
  - Associated pelvic tumors.
– *Gynecology:*
  - Normal pelvic anatomy
  - Uterine size and endometrial thickness
  - Measurement of ovaries
  - Pelvic tumors , e.g. fibroids, cysts, hydrosalpinx
  - Peritoneal fluid
  - Intrauterine contraceptive devices.

- The trainee to be able to recognize the following normal fetal anatomical features from 18 weeks onwards by abdominal ultrasound.
  – *Shape of the skull:* Nuchal skinfold
  – *Brain:* Ventricles and cerebellum, choroid plexus
  – Facial profile
  – *Spine:* Both longitudinally and transversely
  – Heart rate and rhythm, size and position, four-chamber view
  – Size and morphology of the lungs
  – Shape of the thorax and abdomen
  – *Abdomen:* Diaphragm, stomach, liver and umbilical vein, kidneys, abdominal wall and umbilicus
  – Limbs femur, tibia and fibula, humerus, radius and ulna, feet and hands—these to include shape, echogenicity and movement

- – *Multiple pregnancy:* Monochorionic and dischorionic, twin-twin transfusion syndrome
- – Amount of amniotic fluid
- – Placental location
- – Cord and number of vessels.
- Fetal biometry
  - – Crown rump length, biparietal diameter, femur length, head circumference, abdominal circumference, interpretation of growth charts.
- *Activity:* Recognize and quantify
  - – Fetal movements
  - – Breathing movements
  - – Eye movements.

Certification

- One hundred hours of supervised scanning to include:
  - – Hundred gynecological examinations and early pregnancy problems (principally by transvaginal sonography but transabdominal experience also required).
  - – Two hundreds obstetric scans covering the full spectrum of obstetric conditions.
- *Logbooks:* Thirty cases on one A4 page with ultrasound picture, at least 15 anomalies should be included
- *Examination:* General guidelines—the examination would be included as part of the normal obstetrics and gynecology training. The options are to have a multiple-choice paper of short written examination paper (3–4 cases). On the practical side, a transvaginal scan and a fetal anatomy scan, 30 minutes for both, would be recommended. The candidate would take ultrasound pictures and interpret the images.

FOGSI-ICOG Certificate Courses in Obstetrics Gynecology Ultrasonography

Introduction

Ultrasonography is the most commonly used imaging modality in obstetrics and gynecology. Since the popularization of ultrasonography in obstetrics by Professor Ian Donald in the '60s, the diagnostic capability of sonology has improved tremendously especially after the mid '80s. This tremendous improvement of machines over the last ten years has made it the most revolutionizing investigative tool introduced into the practice of obstetrics and gynecology.

Unfortunately, most obstetricians and gynecologists have not kept in the time with the rapid advancement with the diagnostic potential of this equipment. This has lead to obstetric and gynecological use of sonology (80%) as the number one cause of medicolegal litigation in entire sonology. Number one being missed diagnosis of ectopic pregnancy followed by missed diagnosis of congenital malformation. This situation has been primarily due to no clear cut guidelines set up in countries for training of obstetricians in usage of sonology.

Basic Course

Basic training constitutes three days of intensive lectures. The topics have been listed below. Following which, part-time participants have to return to their respective hospitals of origin with logbooks. They are supposed to log a total of four hundred cases (400) over a period of 6 months which includes:
- Forty 1st trimester scans (20 transvaginal scans)
- Two hundreds 2nd trimester scans (follow basic recommendation)
- Forty 3rd trimester scans (follow basic recommendation)
- Sixty cases of normal uterus and ovaries (follow basic recommendation)

- Forty cases of gynecological pathology (follow basic recommendation).

All cases need to be filled in the logbook and the requirement must be completed within maximum of 6 months.

The logbook and the video recording is certified by the training faculty. After that, the candidate to be assessed with patients; which involves one first trimester scan , one second trimester scan , one third trimester scan for growth and fetal assessment and one transvaginal gynecological scan over a period of two hours.

Advanced Course

This entails a few lectures, followed at training center for hands-on experience. Following which, the part-time candidates return to their hospitals of origin with their logbooks. They are supposed to log a total of four hundred (400) cases over a period of 6 months which includes:

- Twenty transvaginal abnormal first trimester scanning least one case for each week up to 2 week for missed abortion, molar pregnancy, ectopic pregnancy.
- Two hundreds cases of detailed anatomical surveillance of a fetus at 22 weeks and after with fetal echocardiography (follow basic requirement given).
- Ten cases of transvaginal fetal abnormality scan at 13–14 weeks (follow basic requirement given).
- Twenty cases of third trimester fetal well-being assessment including growth, amniotic fluid assessment (detailed Doppler assessment, if available) and biophysical profile.
- Fetal abnormalities diagnosed with one case of each major system diagnosed and documented on videotapes or pictures.
- Observation of 10 invasive procedures in obstetrics.
- Observation of 10 cases of Doppler assessment of fetus.

- Hundred cases of transvaginal assess of normal uterus and with or without follicular measurements (at least 20 cases of pathology).
- Observation of 10 cases of color flow imaging and Doppler assessment of gynecological masses.
- Fifteen cases of cyst aspiration or ovum retrieval under ultrasound guidance to be observed.
- To observe 5 cases of hysterosonography with color flow imaging.

All cases done or observed needs to be filled in the logbook and the requirement must be completed within a maximum of six months after commencement, video recording of two of each of the categories for a, b and c and all abnormal conditions (both obstetrics and gynecology) with patient's references number sent to the teaching faculty.

The Logbook and the video-recording must be certified by the teaching faculty. After that, the candidate is sent to teaching faculty to be assessed which would include theory and practical sessions.

Both theory and practical assessments. The theory assessment would mainly involve previewing a total of 30 slides in 40 minutes.

The practical session would involve:

- Early second trimester fetal abnormality scan at 14 weeks
- Detailed fetal abnormality scan at 22 weeks and after with fetal echocardiography
- Transvaginal assessment of pelvic anatomy
- One third trimester scan to assess fetal well-being
  All these to be completed in 1½ hours.

If the categorizing of cases in the logbook, video-casette recordings and clinical assessment are all satisfactory, then the candidate will be a certificate in issued ultrasonography in obstetrics by ICOG-FOGSI.

Antenatal Diagnostic Center, Department of Obstetrics and Gynecology

Guidelines for Repeat Obstetric Ultrasonography for Fetal Growth

- Fetal number, lie, presentation, FH and FM
- Amount of amniotic fluid
    - Excessive, normal/decreased
    - (Amniotic fluid index-AFI)
    - If abnormal AFI.
- AC-95th/75th/50th/25th/5th percentile for data EFW in grams, no other measurements necessary if AC is between 75th and 25th percentile
- (PRN) HC/AC ratio {If AC is below 25th or FL/AC ratio} above 75th percentiles, repeat scan 3 to 4 weekly interval from 28 weeks
    - If liquor volume decreased
    - AC is < 5th percentile
    - or abnormal H/S or FL/AC ratio.

Antenatal Fetal Monitoring for High Risk Pregnancy

Verify date by first trimester vE

or

U/S 18 or 20 weeks

Serial SFH from 2nd trimester length of a new needed FMC by mother from 3rd trimester U/S growth assessment 28–30 weeks repeat 32–34 weeks

Normal U/S Growth	Decreased U/S Growth
Weekly CTG from 34 weeks, if liquor is decreased	i. CTG biweekly/3 per week Biophysical profile weekly ii. Serial 3 to 4 weekly U/S growth from 28 weeks iii. Blood flow studies weekly

Suggested Scheme for Ultrasonic Scanning

General scanning for ALL cases
- Number of fetuses
- Lie and presentation
- Liquor volume: Excessive/normal
  - Qualitative assessment: Decreased
  - Quantitative assessment (depth and width)
- Placenta-Location
  - Grade (0–III)
  - Abnormalities
  - Retroplacental space
- Membranes
- Cord-vessels.
- Systemic screening for fetal anomalies
- Head - BPD, HC
  - OFD, OFD/BPD ratio
  - Anterior and posterior V/H ratio
  - Thalamic and mid-brain view
  - Cerebral peduncle view
  - Cerebellar view, transverse cerebellar diameter
  - Ocular view and diameters
  - Base of skull, hard palate
  - Integrity of skull table, encephalocele
  - Face and lips
- Neck: Soft tissue swelling
- Spine: Cervical region
  - Thoracic region
  - Lumbosacral region
    - Longitudinal view
    - Transverse view
    - Lateral view.
  - Each region
- Chest
  - Pleural effusion

- – Pericardial effusion
- – Long parenchyma
- – Chest circumference
- – Heart
  - - Four chamber view
  - - Left ventricular view
  - - Right ventricular view
  - - Short axis view
  - - Aortic root view
  - - Pulmonary root view
  - - TM studies
- Diaphragm
  - – Herniation of guts
- Abdomen
  - – Presence of ascites
  - – Abdominal wall, cord insertion
  - – Stomach
  - – Liver, umbilical veins
  - – AC
  - – Kidneys
    - - Appearance
    - - Size (KC, KC/AC ratio)
    - - Renal pelvis, ureter
  - – Bladder, genitalia
  - – Bowel distension
- Extremities
  - – Femur, tibia and fibula, humerus, radius and ulna
  - – Fingers and toes
  - – Degree of skeletal calcification
  - – Femur/BPD ratio
- Soft tissues
  - – Subcutaneous thickness
  - – Swelling/edema

- Fetal behavior
  - Swallowing
  - Limb movements
  - Body tone

Screening for IUGR
- BPD and HC
- AC
- H/A ratio
- Femur/AC ratio
- CRL TA
- TIUV
- Thigh thickness/femur length
- Estimated fetal weight and FW zone

  Comment on as symmetrical IUGR: Screen for fetal well-being.

  Repeat every 3 to 4 weeks during 3rd trimester (from weeks onwards).

Screening for fetal well-being
- Biophysical profile and score
  - FM
  - BM
  - Tone
  - AFV
  - CTG

  Repeat twice a week for diabetes, IUGR and post-term.

  Once a week for maternal/physician concern, decreased fetal movement and other high-risk conditions.

Blood flow studies for growth retarded fetus.

Basic Principles of Medical Ultrasound

- The relevant principles of acoustics, attenuation, absorption, reflection, speed to sound
- The effect on tissues of pulsed and continuous wave ultrasound beams: biological effects, thermal and nonthermal

- Basic operating principles of medical instruments:
  - Pulse echo, scanning principles and 3D
  - Pulse echo instruments, including linear array, curvilinear, mechanical sector, transvaginal and rectal scanners
  - Velocity imaging and recording:
    - Doppler principle
    - Continuous wave
      » Pulse wave
      » Color flow mapping
      » Power Doppler
    - Color velocity imaging
    - Pitfalls, artifacts
  - Data acquisition
  - Signal processing (may be given in practical demonstration):
    - Gray scale
    - Time gain compensation
    - Dynamic range
    - Dynamic focus
    - Gain compensation, acoustic output relationship (may be given in practical demonstration)
  - Artefacts, interpretation and avoidance
    - Reverberation
    - Side lobes
    - Edge effects
    - Registration
    - Shadowing
    - Enhancement
  - Measuring systems
    - Linear, circumference, area and volume
    - Doppler ultrasound-flow, velocity spectrum analysis
  - Imaging recording, storage and analysis
  - Interpretation of acoustic output information and its clinical relevance.

Obstetrics

- Investigation of early pregnancy:
  - Ultrasound features of normal early pregnancy, including gestational sac and yolk sac, simple and multiple pregnancy, chorionicity
  - Development of fetal anatomy in early pregnancy including recognition of abnormalities, such as nuchal translucency, cystic hygroma and fetal hydrops
  - Embryonic-fetal biometry, e.g. crown-rump length
  - Fetal viability
  - Ultrasound features of early pregnancy failure including hydatidiform mole
  - Ultrasound and biochemical investigation of ectopic pregnancy
  - Normal appearance of the cervix
- Assessment of amniotic fluid and placenta:
  - Estimation of amniotic fluid volume
  - Examination of the placenta and cord
  - Placental location
  - Number of cord vessels
- Normal fetal anatomy at 18–22 weeks:
  - Shape of skull: Nuchal fold
  - Facial profile
  - *Brain:* Cerebral ventricles, posterior fossa and cerebellum; cisterna magna, choroid plexus cysts
  - *Spine:* Both longitudinally and transversely
  - Heart rate and rhythm, four-chamber view, including atrioventricular valves, outflow tract
  - Lungs
  - Shape of the thorax and abdomen
  - *Abdomen:* Stomach, liver, kidneys and urinary bladder, abdominal wall and umbilicus

- – *Limbs:* Femur, tibia and fibula, humerus, radius and ulna, hands and feet-these to include shape and echogenicity of the long bones and movement
  - – *Multiple pregnancy:* Chorionicity
- To study the epidemiology, differential diagnosis, natural history of abnormalities and management of:
  - – Structural
    - - Skeletal system
    - - Central nervous system
    - - Cardiovascular
    - - lntrathoracic disorders
    - - Renal
    - - Abdominal wall and diaphragm
    - - Gastrointestinal
    - - Markers for chromosomal abnormalities
  - – Functional
    - - Polyhydramnios, oligohydramnios, hydrops, dysrhythmias
  - – Prognosis and treatment (including intravascular therapy)
- Fetal biometry:
  - – Measurements to assess fetal size (including biparietal diameter, head circumference, abdominal circumference, femur length)
  - – Measurements to aid the diagnosis of fetal anomalies; anterior/posterior horn of the lateral ventricle, transcerebellar diameter, nuchal skinfold
- Estimation of gestational age:
  - – Interpretation and appreciation of limitation of ultrasonic and other investigations for gestational age assessment
- Assessment of fetal growth:
  - – Ultrasonic assessment of fetal growth interpretation and appreciation of limitations of standard measurements singly or serially
  - – Fetal weight estimation

- Biophysical scoring systems: Interpretation and appreciation of limitations:
  - Fetal body movements
  - Fetal breathing
  - Heart rate and rhythm
- Evaluation of fetal and uteroplacental blood flow:
  - Methodology appropriate to obstetric investigation
  - Appreciation of problems in blood flow and velocity measurements and waveform analysis in normal and complicated pregnancies
  - Clinical applications and limitations in the prediction of intrauterine growth retardation and pre-eclampsia
  - Clinical applications in monitoring the small for dates fetus and pregnancies complicated by rhesus isoimmunization, diabetes and fetal cardiac arrhythmias
- Knowledge of invasive diagnostic and therapeutic procedures:
  - *Diagnostic:* Amniocentesis, chorionic sampling, cordocentesis
  - *Therapeutic:* Shunting and draining procedures.

Gynecology

- Normal pelvic anatomy:
  - Uterus
    - Uterine size, position, shape and movement
    - Cyclical morphological changes in the endometrium
    - Measurement of endometrial thickness
  - Ovaries
    - Size, position, shape and measurement
    - Cyclical morphological changes
    - Measurement of follicles and corpus luteum
    - Assessment of peritoneal fluid
- Gynecological complications:
  - Uterus

- - Fibroids
  - Adenomyosis
  - Endometrial hyperplasia
  - Endometrial cancer
  - Polyps
  - Location of intrauterine contraceptive device
- Tubes
  - Hydrosalpinx and other abnormalities of the fallopian tubes
- Ovaries
  - Cysts; benign and malignant, morphological scoring systems
  - Endometriosis
  - Ovarian carcinoma
  - Differential diagnosis of pelvic masses.
- Infertility:
  - Monitoring of follicular development in spontaneous and stimulated cycles
    - Diagnosis of hyperstimulation syndrome
    - Diagnosis of polycystic ovaries
    - Sonosalpingography.
- Invasive procedures:
  - Oocyte retrieval
  - Injection of ovarian cysts
  - Aspiration of ovarian cysts
  - Drainage of pelvic abscesses
  - Extraction of intrauterine contraceptive device;
- Doppler in gynecology
  - Infertility and oncology

Organization of Ultrasound Unit

Infrastructure, documentation, quality control, computerization and data storage.

Medicolegal Implications of Ultrasound Examination Ethics and Patient Information

Practical training: Required skills

- The trainee to be able to identify early pregnancy and emergency gynecological problems by transvaginal and transabdominal ultrasound.
    - Early pregnancy
        - Fetal viability
        - Description of the gestational sac, embryo and yolk sac
        - Single and multiple gestation (chorionicity).
    - Pathology
        - Early pregnancy failure
        - Ectopic pregnancy
        - Gross fetal abnormalities, such as nuchal translucency, hydropic abnormalities
        - Hydatidiform mole
        - Associated pelvic tumors.
    - Gynecology
        - Normal pelvic anatomy
        - Uterine size and endometrial thickness
        - Measurement of ovaries
        - Pelvic tumors, e.g., fibroids, cysts, hydrosalpinx
        - Peritoneal fluid
        - Intrauterine contraceptive devices.
- The trainee should be able to recognize the following normal fetal anatomical features from 18 weeks onwards by abdominal ultrasound.
    - Shape of the skull; nuchal fold
    - Brain: Ventricles and cerebellum, chorid plexus
    - Facial profile

- *Spine:* Both longitudinally and transversely
- Heart rate and rhythm, size and position, four-chamber view
- Size and morphology and of the lungs
- Shape of the thorax and abdomen
- *Abdomen:* Diaphragm, stomach, liver and umbilical vein, kidneys, abdominal wall and umbilicus
- *Limbs:* Femur, tibia and fibula, humerus, radiums and ulna, feet and hands these to include shape, echogenicity and movement
- *Multiple pregnancy:* Monochorionic and dichorionic, twin to twin transfusion syndrome
- Amount of amniotic fluid
- Placental location
- Cord and number of vessels
- *Fetal biometry:*
  - Crown-rump length, biparietal diameter, femur length, head circumference, abdominal circumference, interpretation of growth charts
- *Activity:* Recognize and quantify:
  - Fetal movement
  - Breathing movements
  - Eye movements.

There can be maximum 2 ICOG delegates for ultrasonography course training at any one time in a given center.

Evaluation

The evaluation of learning outcome of trainees consists of:

Assessment plan during the course:
There will be continuous monitoring and regular assessment of all academic activities of the candidate.

Formal evaluation is done by the staff of the department based on participation of students in various teaching/learning activities. The evaluation is structured on the basis of checklists that evaluate these various parameters.

The following aspects will be assessed:

- *Personal attitudes:* It is pertinent to assess and guide the candidate in facing stressful conditions in the ward and operating room, to assess the candidate's ability to work as a team and to evaluate the leadership qualities, and coordinating abilities.
- *Acquisition of knowledge:* This will be done by evaluation of the candidate's performance during the journal club, seminars, symposia, interactive conferences and discussions during the ward rounds.

CHECK-LIST FOR EVALUATION OF SEMINAR PRESENTATIONS

Parameters evaluated	Poor (0)	Below average (1)	Average (2)	Good (3)	Very good (4)
1. Relevant publications consulted					
2. Cross-references consulted					
3. Completeness of preparation					
4. Clarity of presentation					
5. Understanding of subject					
6. Ability of answer questions					
7. Time scheduling					
8. Audio-visual aids					
9. Overall performance					
10. Overall quality of ward work					

CHECK-LIST FOR EVALUATION OF CLINICAL WORK

Parameters evaluated	Poor (0)	Below average (1)	Average (2)	Good (3)	Very good (4)
1. Regularity of attendance					
2. Punctuality					
3. Interaction with colleagues					
4. Maintenance of case records					
5. Case presentation during					
6. Investigations work up					
7. Bedside manners					
8. Rapport with patients					
9. Counseling patient's relatives					
10. Overall quality of ward work					

Logbook

Prime importance will be given to maintaining a proper record of events of teaching and experiences that the candidate has obtained in a log book. Internal assessment will be based on the evaluation of the log book. The record will include academic activities as well as the presentations and procedures carried out by the candidate.

Assessment for Certification

Eligibility: The teacher certifies the candidate's competence and performance, the ICOG-FOGSI will grant permission for assessment.

The written assessment: There shall be a written assessment at the end consisting of at least two question papers. Each paper shall carry 100 marks. One paper of MCQs and 2nd of 5–6 short questions.

Practical Examination: There shall be one external examiner, generally by an external examiner appointed by the ICOG-FOGSI. One hour, maximum 100 marks.

Certification: Based on the recommendations made by the examiners, successful candidate would be awarded the certificate scroll by ICOG-FOGSI. In case of unsatisfactory completion, the trainee would be given another chance to appear before the examination (6 months) later.

Fee Structure

The candidate will be asked to pay ₹50,000 by demand draft in favor of FOGSI with prescribed application form selecting a center to the ICOG-FOGSI at the time of admission toward the fee for the ICOG-FOGSI Certificate course in ultrasonography.

The institution will not collect any fee from the candidates. No stipend will be paid to the trainee.

Criteria for Selection

The candidate applying for certificate course in gynecological endoscopic and minimal access surgery should have successfully completed:

- MD/DGO/FCPS in Obstetrics and Gynecology in MCI approved place or DNB in Obstetrics and Gynecology in NBE approved place
- Should be an active member of FOGSI Society.

Accommodation Facilities

At present there is no accommodation facility given at the institution for the trainees. The trainee is required to make his/her arrangements for accommodation.

Introduction

3.1 FILLING UP OF FORMS

Maintain a form for further follow-up in your clinic. One never knows when the information is required.

The routine information required in these forms is:

- Name
- Age
- Address
- Telephone number
- Referred by
- PNDT Act Form 'F' as required by Government of India Law
- Undertaking by patient and doctor for obstetric ultrasound with Form 'F'.

3.2 RELEVANT HISTORY

Always spend few minutes with your patient to take the details of the history. Gives confidence to the patient and you get your perspective of what all to expect. The history to be taken routinely is:

- Previous obstetric history consisting of details of any abortions (spontaneous or missed), any second or third trimester losses (possible reasons), any previous deliveries (vaginal or cesarean). Try and look into the previous records which can throw any light.
- Any symptoms in this pregnancy
- Any ultrasound done so far in this pregnancy. Check the records carefully.
- Last menstrual period and regularity of menstrual cycles.
- Any tests done and their reports.
- Referring doctor requisition slip along with registration and stamp. This is now a legal requirement with Form 'F'.

3.3 PREPARATION AND POSITIONING OF PATIENT

- In scans up to 15 weeks a full bladder is required, unless transvaginal. It is preferable to examine up to 12 weeks by a transvaginal scan.
- Between 15 and 22 weeks holding urine for 1 hour is sufficient.
- After 22 weeks no preparation is required. A full bladder for assessment of the cervix and lower segment assessment can be asked for when required.
- The patient need not be fasting unless and until an upper abdomen scan is also asked for.
- The patient is almost always scanned supine with plenty of jelly on the abdomen. In certain cases scanning in the lateral position (if patient is uncomfortable lying supine or fetus moves when lying in a lateral position) or with the patient standing (for functional assessment of cervix) is required.

- Whenever, a transvaginal scan is asked for the bladder must be emptied immediately before the examination. It should be performed with the same respect for privacy and gentleness, as is with the placement of a speculum. Scanning is performed with the patient supine and with her thighs abducted and knees flexed. Elevation of the buttock may be necessary. The probe should be covered with a condom or sheath containing a small amount of gel. Additional gel should be placed on the outside of sheathed tip. The probe is inserted by a gentle push posteriorly toward the rectum while the patient relaxes.

Four types of probe movements are required:
  - Pushing and pulling
  - Rotation
  - "Rocking" or upward and downward
  - Side-to-side or "Panning".

After removal of the transvaginal probe, the sheath is removed and the coupling gel is wiped off with a damp towel. The TV probe may be disinfected by Cidex.

3.4 MACHINE AND TRANSDUCERS

- For a transabdominal scan, a 3.5–5.0 MHz transducer and for a transvaginal scan, a 5.0–8.0 MHz transducer is used.
- Basic controls of every machine are more or less the same. The placement of knobs is different for all machines. Check for the manual of your machine or somebody from the company can always come and explain you.

The routine Knobology is:
  - Patient's name and entry of last menstrual period after you select the obstetric mode
  - Freeze
  - B, B + B, B + M or only M mode
  - Depth and focus
  - Overall gain
  - Time gain (TGC)

- Comments on screen
- Measurement (set and select) for linear, area, and volume
- Track ball or screen or joy stick to move the cursor
- Color flow map, power Doppler, Doppler and 3D and 4D.
- After freezing the images these can be stored and a print taken on a camera, thermal printer or from a computer.

3.5 REPORTING

Maximum possible information to be given in the report to the patient.

Routinely four ultrasounds should be asked for in all pregnancies. The parameters to be checked in all four ultrasounds are mentioned. They are:

From 6 to 9 Weeks

- Uterine size manual (7.5 cm length, 5 cm wide, 2.5 cm thickness)
- Location of gestational sac
- Number of gestational sacs
- Size of gestational sac
- Yolk sac/No of yolk sac
- Size of yolk sac
- Embryo/fetus size
- Menstrual age
- Cardiac activity (±)
- Heart rate
- Trophoblastic reaction
- Any uterine mass
- Any adnexal mass
- Corpus luteum (present/absent)
- Subchorionic hematoma

From 10 to 14 Weeks

- Placental site
- Liquor amnii
- Fetal crown rump length
- Menstrual age
- Fetal movements and cardiac activity
- Any gross anomalies
- Nuchal translucency
- Nasal bone (present/absent)
- Ductus venosus flow
- Internal os width
- Length of cervix
- Any uterine mass
- Any adnexal mass.

From 18 to 22 Weeks

- Placenta
  - Heart-Portion-four chamber outflow tract
- Liquor amnii
- Umbilical cord
- Cervix
- Lower segment
  - Internal OS
- Myometrium
- Adnexa
- Nuchal skin thickness
- Cerebellar transverse diameter
- Cisterna magna depth
- Width of body of lateral ventricle
- Inter-hemispheric distance
- Ratio of the width of body of lateral ventricle to inter-hemispheric distance
- Ocular diameter

- Interocular distance
- Binocular distance
- Biparietal diameter
- Occipitofrontal distance
- Head perimeter
- Abdominal perimeter
- Femoral length
- Humeral length
- Foot length
- Fetal movements and cardiac activity
- Ductus venosus flow velocity waveform
- Both maternal uterine artery Doppler
- Presence of all organs and any abnormality detected

From 35 to 40 Weeks

- Placenta
- Liquor amnii
- Umbilical cord
- Cervix
- Lower segment
- Myometrium
- Adnexa
- Biparietal diameter
- Occipitofrontal distance
- Head perimeter
- Abdominal perimeter
- Femoral length
- Distal femoral epiphysis
- Biophysical profile/modified biophysical profile (AFI and VAST)
- Color Doppler arterial (umbilical artery, middle cerebral artery, descending aorta and both maternal uterine arteries)
- Color Doppler venous (umbilical vein, inferior vena cava and ductus venosus).

4

First Trimester

4·1 INDICATIONS

- Confirmation of pregnancy
- Vaginal bleeding in pregnancy (threatened abortion)
- Estimation of gestational age
- Suspected ectopic pregnancy
- Suspected hydatidiform mole
- Adjunct to cervical cerclage
- Suspected multiple gestation
- Adjunct to chorionic villus sampling.

4.2 NORMAL FIRST TRIMESTER EMBRYONIC/FETAL EVALUATION

- Location of sac:
  - Fundus (Fig. 4.1)
  - Corpus (Fig. 4.2)
  - Cornual (Fig. 4.3)
  - Superior to the cervix.
- Number of sacs:
  - Single
  - Multiple (Twin/triplet/high order multiple) (Fig. 4.4).
- Size of sac:

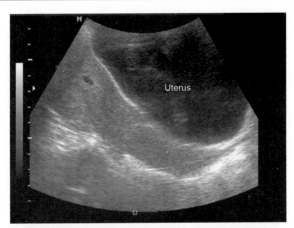

Fig. 4.1: Gestational sac located in the uterine fundus.

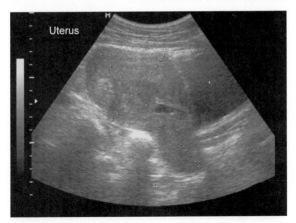

Fig. 4.2: Gestational sac located in the uterine corpus.

– In toto, measure inner to inner diameter of gestational sac on all three sides and calculate the size and corresponding gestational age (Figs. 4.5A and B)

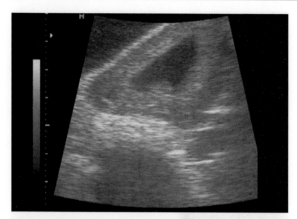

Fig. 4.3: Gestational sac located in the uterine cavity in the cornual area. Note the amount of myometrium lateral to the gestational sac differentiating it from a cornual ectopic.

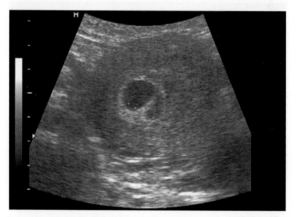

Fig. 4.4: Two gestational sacs both located in the uterine fundus.

- – Size of gestational sac in comparison to the embryo/fetus size (Fig. 4.6).
- • Embryo/fetal size (crown rump length) (Figs. 4.7 and 4.8).

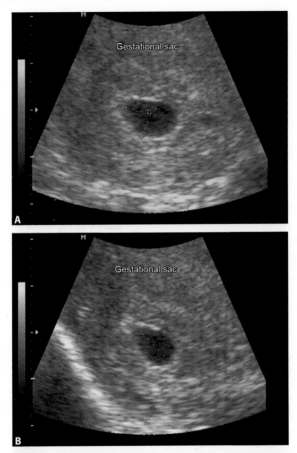

Figs. 4.5A and B: Gestational sac measurement in all three planes and calculation of gestational age done by the ultrasound machine.

- Embryonic cardiac activity. To begin with, the heart rate is around 85 beats/minute at 5 to 5½ weeks (Fig. 4.9) increasing to around 160 beats/minute (Fig. 4.10) at nine weeks.
- Yolk sac:

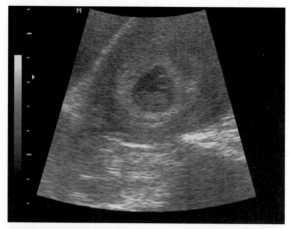

Fig. 4.6: Note that the sac is oligoamniotic with the gestational sac corresponding less than the embryo size.

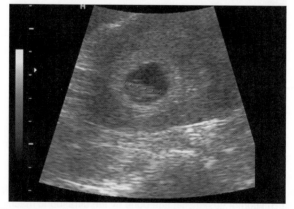

Fig. 4.7: Measurement of crown rump length in a 7 weeks and 6 days embryo.

- Size
- Shape
- Any calcification.

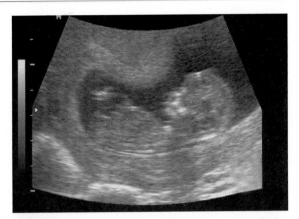

Fig. 4.8: Measurement of crown rump length in an 12 weeks and 4 days fetus.

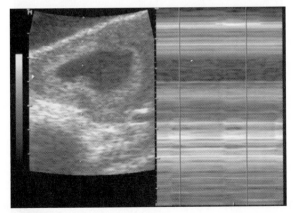

Fig. 4.9: Heart rate of 143 beats per minute in a 6 weeks and 0 day embryo.

- Trophoblastic reaction:
    - Whether wrapping around and thick reaction (Fig. 4.11)
    - Locate site (Fig. 4.12).

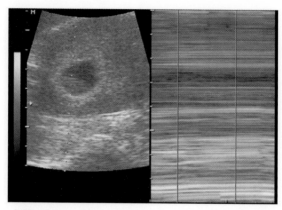

Fig. 4.10: Heart rate of 151 beats per minute in an 8 weeks and 1 day fetus.

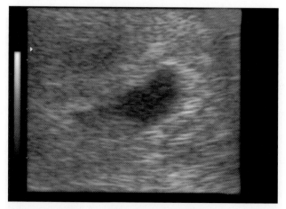

Fig. 4.11: Wrapping around thick trophoblastic reaction seen in a gestational sac of 6 weeks 4 days.

- Separation:
  - Amniodecidual separation (Fig. 4.13)
  - Choriodecidual separation (Fig. 4.14).
- To identify any gross anomalies:

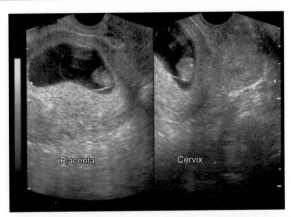

Fig. 4.12: Note the thickened trophoblastic echoes on one wall of the gestational sac. This is the placental site location.

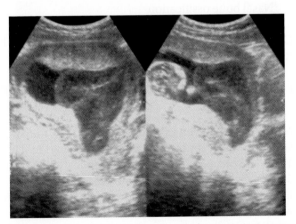

Fig. 4.13: The placenta is anterior with an amniodecidual separation seen in the anterior wall superior to the cervix. This has an associated collection of 8.35 mL.

– Gross abnormalities of the cranium, spine, abdomen and limbs can be detected even in the late first trimester

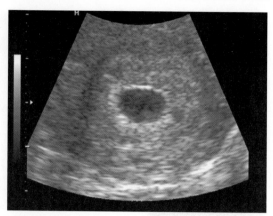

Fig. 4.14: Multiple foci of choriodecidual separation seen in a 6–7 weeks size missed abortion.

- Nasal bone ossification
- Nuchal translucency.
- Color Doppler evaluation of the ductus venosus and both maternal uterine arteries.

4.3 NORMAL PARAMETER EVALUATION IN THE FIRST TRIMESTER

- *Gestational sac:* Seen as early as 4½ weeks by transvaginal scan and 5½ weeks by transabdominal scan (Fig. 4.15).
- *Yolk sac:* Seen as early as 5 weeks by transvaginal scan and 6 weeks by transabdominal scan (Fig. 4.16).
- *Embryo:* Seen at 5½ weeks by transvaginal scan and at 6–6½ weeks by transabdominal scan (Fig. 4.17).
- *Cardiac activity:* Appears at 5 weeks and 4 days.

4.4 ABNORMAL INTRAUTERINE PREGNANCY

- No embryonic cardiac activity with a CRL >5 mm. (missed abortion) (Fig. 4.18)

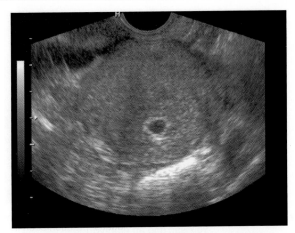

Fig. 4.15: Transvaginal scan of a gestational sac of 5 weeks size.

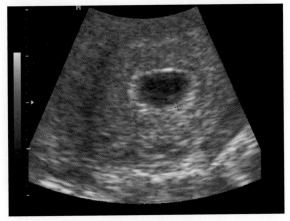

Fig. 4.16: Gestational sac of 5 weeks and 2 days with a yolk sac clearly delineated.

- Gestational sac larger than 8 mm without a yolk sac. (blighted ovum) (Fig. 4.19).

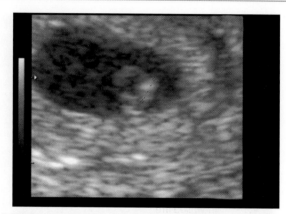

Fig. 4.17: Pregnancy of 5 weeks and 6 days gestation showing a yolk sac and an embryo.

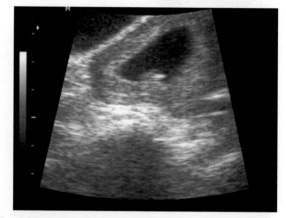

Fig. 4.18: No cardiac activity seen in this 8 mm pulseless attenuated embryo.

- Gestational sac larger than 16 mm without an embryo. (anembryonic pregnancy) (Fig. 4.20).
- Abnormally large or irregular or small amniotic sac (Fig. 4.21).

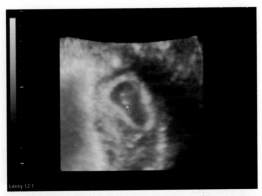

Fig. 4.19: Thin-walled irregular gestational sac of 15 mm in the uterine fundus with a pulseless embryo.

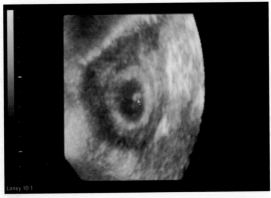

Fig. 4.20: Seven weeks gestational sac showing a yolk sac but no embryo.

4.5 IMPENDING EARLY PREGNANCY FAILURE

- Embryonic bradycardia relative to CRL.
- Mean sac diameter minus CRL is less than 5 mm (oligoamniotic sac).

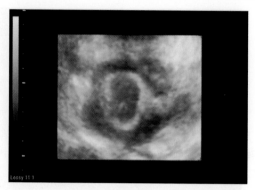

Fig. 4.21: Large, flaccid and irregular amniotic sac with a
pulseless embryo.

- Poor sac growth
- Large (> 5.6 mm prior to 10 weeks)/abnormal yolk sac
  (Figs. 4.22 and 4.23).
- Disappearance of the corpus luteum.

Classification of Early Pregnancy Loss (Tables 4.1 and 4.2)

Stage A:
- Loss within first 2 weeks
- Subclinical loss
- No sonographic evidence.

Stage B:
- Loss at 5–6 weeks
- Empty gestational sac.

Stage C:
- Loss at 7–8 weeks
- Abnormal gestational sac and embryo.

Stage D:
- Loss at 9–12 weeks
- Abnormal embryo.

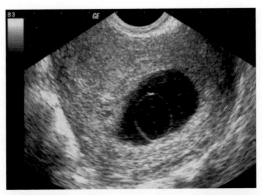

Fig. 4.22: Large yolk sac with the embryo seen adjacent to it.

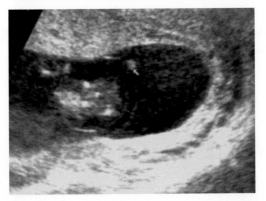

Fig. 4.23: Shrunken yolk sac with an extensive cystic hygroma associated with it.

4.6 ECTOPIC GESTATION

- Demonstration of live embryo in the adnexa is diagnostic of ectopic pregnancy (Fig. 4.24).
- Nonspecific findings of an ectopic pregnancy are an adnexal mass, free fluid (Fig. 4.25), a tubal ring (Fig. 4.26)

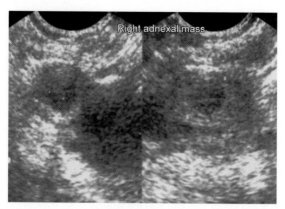

Fig. 4.24: Live ectopic with a gestational sac, yolk sac and an embryo with cardiac activity.

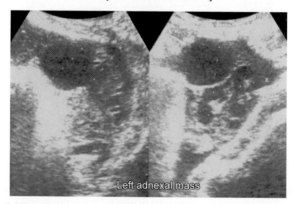

Fig. 4.25: Left adnexal mass with corpus luteum in the left ovary with an adjacent inhomogeneous adnexal mass and perilesional fluid collection.

and identification of adnexal peritrophoblastic flow (Fig. 4.27).

- Vascular ring can be delineated (Fig. 4.28).
- The blood flow characteristically shows low-impedance, high-diastolic flow.

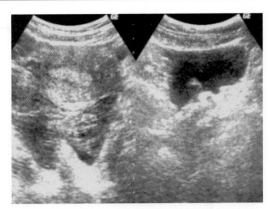

Fig. 4.26: Adnexal mass with free fluid (pelvic hematocele) in the pouch of Douglas.

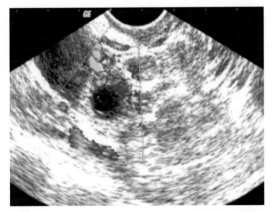

Fig. 4.27: On color Doppler in an ectopic pregnancy which is unruptured with viable trophoblasts a vascular ring is delineated with the blood flow characteristically showing low-impedance, high-diastolic flow.

- Intrauterine peritrophoblastic flow is not seen and periendometrial venous flow is also very less.
- Corpus luteal flow is identified in one or both ovaries.

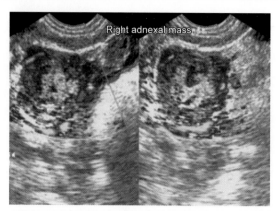

Fig. 4.28: Same case with marked peritrophoblastic vascularity in the mass.

4.7 EXTRA-FETAL EVALUATION

- Myometrium (Fig. 4.29)
- Cervical length (Fig. 4.30)
- Internal os
- Adnexal mass (Fig. 4.31)
- Site of corpus luteum (Fig. 4.32)
- Vascularity of corpus luteum (Figs. 4.33 and 4.34).

4.8 ABNORMAL INTRAUTERINE PREGNANCY FORMS

- Threatened/missed abortion
- Incomplete abortion
- Complete abortion
- Hydatiform mole
- Blighted ovum.

4.9 COMPLETE ABORTION

- No intrauterine gestational sac seen (empty uterus sign)
- Cavity echoes are thin and usually homogeneous (Fig. 4.35)

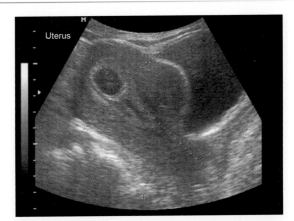

Fig. 4.29: Look for any masses in the myometrium. Early pregnancy with a posterior wall subserous fibroid. If you locate any fibroid specify the site (uterine or cervical) and the type (submucous, interstitial, subserous or panmural) so as to assess later in serial scans.

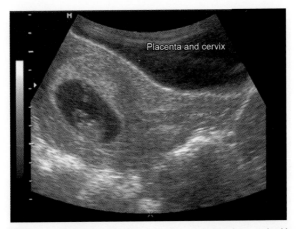

Fig. 4.30: Even in the first trimester always evaluate the cervical length by measuring from the cervical waist or the location of the internal os till the portion where the mucus plug ends. Any herniation or shortening to be reported for serial evaluation.

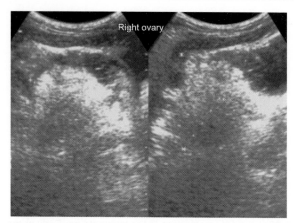

Fig. 4.31: Apart from the corpus luteum always evaluate the adnexa for any masses like dermoid, broad ligament fibroid or any other ovarian masses.

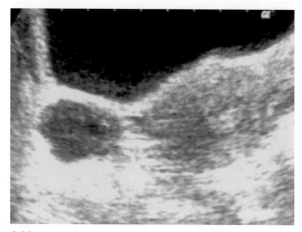

Fig. 4.32: Locate the corpus luteum as to which ovary it is in. Corpus luteum can appear iso- or hypoechoic within the ovary depending on hemorrhage.

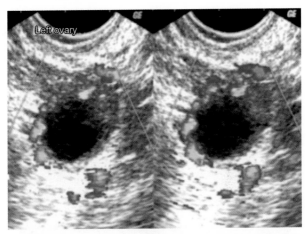

Fig. 4.33: On color flow mapping one can assess the vascularity of the corpus luteum.

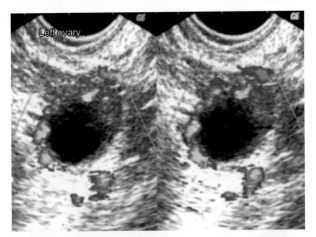

Fig. 4.34: Evaluate the vascularity of the corpus luteum by color flow mapping and the arterial flow velocity waveform on duplex Doppler should normally show a resistive index of less than 0.55.

- Uterine vascularity is cold or warm (Fig. 4.36)
- There is minimal or absent intrauterine peri-trophoblastic flow (Fig. 4.37)
- Intrauterine venous flow is minimal or absent.

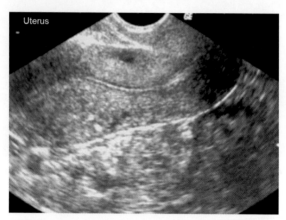

Fig. 4.35: A case of complete spontaneous abortion with very thin cavity echoes, 3–4 mm.

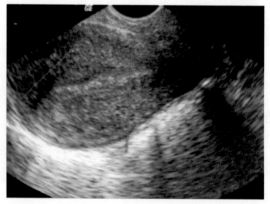

Fig. 4.36: The uterine vascularity is usually cold in a case of complete spontaneous abortion.

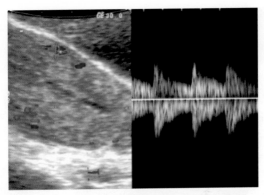

Fig. 4.37: Intrauterine peritrophoblastic flow is not seen and only peripheral myometrial vascularity seen.

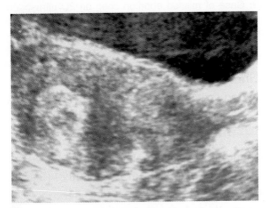

Fig. 4.38: Inhomogeneous echoes within the uterine cavity seen on 2D ultrasound in a case of amenorrhea 6 weeks with bleeding for 3 days.

4.10 INCOMPLETE ABORTION

- Inhomogeneous cavity echoes (Fig. 4.38)
- Overall uterine vascularity diffusely increased (warm or hot vascularity) (Fig. 4.39)

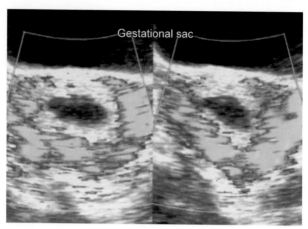

Fig. 4.39: Case of missed abortion seen on 2D ultrasound and on color Doppler, the overall uterine vascularity is increased (warm or hot vascularity).

- Peritrophoblastic arterial flow present with high systolic velocities (Fig. 4.40)
- Periendometrial venous flow also increased (Fig. 4.41).

4.11 MOLAR CHANGE

- Echogenic tissue interspersed with numerous punctate sonolucencies (snow storm appearance) (Figs. 4.42 and 4.43).
- In uncomplicated cases only mild increase in peri-lesional vascularity is noted.
- In invasive moles very high velocity flow in areas of tumor invasion within the myometrium are seen (Fig. 4.44).
- Very low impedance flow with almost an arteriovenous shunt type waveform is also seen.
- Hypervascularity recedes with regression of the tumor.

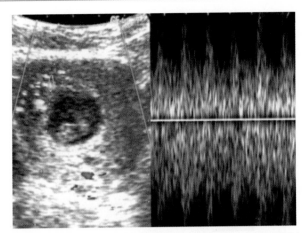

Fig. 4.40: Same case on duplex Doppler evaluation the peritrophoblastic arterial flow is identified, with systolic velocities much above the normal range for intrauterine pregnancy.

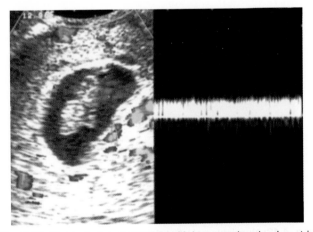

Fig. 4.41: Case of missed abortion with increased periendometrial venous flow.

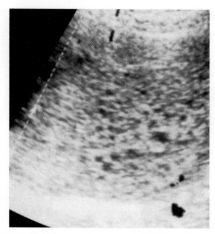

Fig. 4.42: Characteristic cystic spaces packed in the uterine cavity are seen in this case of molar pregnancy.

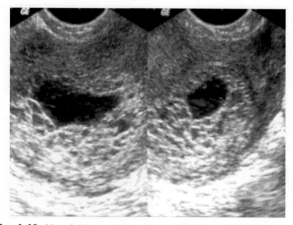

Fig. 4.43: Nonviable gestational sac with thin-walled clear cystic spaces around the gestational sac.

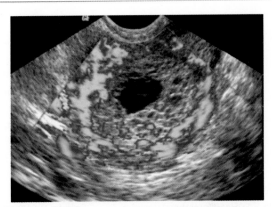

Fig. 4.44: In molar pregnancy in uncomplicated cases only mild increase in perilesional vascularity is noted. In invasive moles very high velocity flow in areas of tumor invasion within the myometrium are seen. Very low impedance flow with almost an arteriovenous shunt type waveform is also seen. This hypervascularity recedes with regression of the tumor.

4.12 SONOEMBRYOLOGY CHART (FIGS. 4.45 TO 4.55)

Date	Event	Sonological evaluation
Day 14	Ovulation Secretory endometrium	Collapse of follicle, free fluid corpus luteum
Day 15	Fertilization	—
Day 18	Morula stage	Decidualization of endometrium
Day 22–23	Blastocyst	Implantation window
Day 23	Primary yolk sac	Implantation site
Day 26–28	Extra-embryonic coelom	Implantation site recognition
Day 27–28	Secondary yolk sac	
Day 28	Syncytiotrophoblast and sometimes seen Chorionic cavity	

Contd...

Contd...

Date	Event	Sonological evaluation
Week 5 29/30	Gastrulation secondary, yolk sac	Visualization of gestational sac, and
31/42	Neuralization	Growth of sac embryo Fetal cardiac activity
34/44	Somites	Embryo visualization Crown rump length Cardiac activity
Week 6–12	Cardiovascular system	—
6 weeks	Unidirectional blood flow	Cardiac activity
8 weeks 10 weeks	Heart/peripheral vascular system	Seen by TVS Visualized
Gastrointestinal tract		
6 weeks	Primitive gut	
8–12 weeks	Gut lies outside in umbilical cord	Physiological herniation
Genitourinary		
8 weeks	Primitive kidney	Not yet seen
11 weeks	Kidney develops urine production	Bladder seen
14 weeks	External genitalia	Can be seen
Musculoskeletal system		
6 weeks	Limb buds	Can be seen
8 weeks	Digital rays clavical ossification	Can be seen Seen
9 weeks	Mandible ossification	Seen
10 weeks	Nasal bone ossification	Seen
10 weeks	Spinal ossification	Spine seen
11 weeks	Frontal bones	
11 Weeks	Long bone ossification	

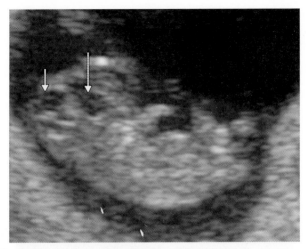

Fig. 4.45: Anechoic areas (arrows) seen in the brain of a fetus of 9 weeks and 6 days.

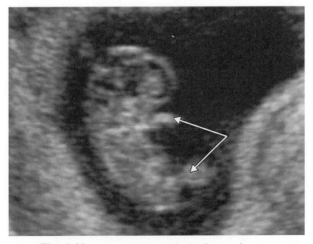

Fig. 4.46: Upper and lower limbs (arrows) seen.

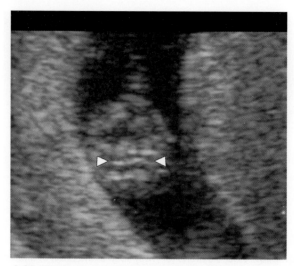

Fig. 4.47: Cerebellar hemispheres (arrowheads) with deficiency in the vermis (physiological at this stage).

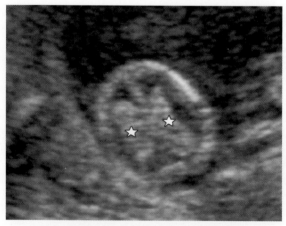

Fig. 4.48: Echogenic choroid plexii (stars) in the lateral ventricles.

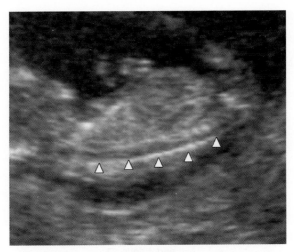

Fig. 4.49: Fetal spine (arrowheads) can be seen as two parallel lines.

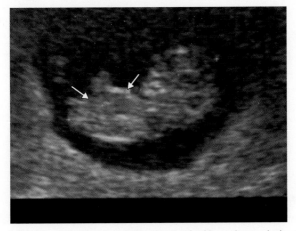

Fig. 4.50: Physiological herniation (arrows) of bowel seen below the umbilical cord.

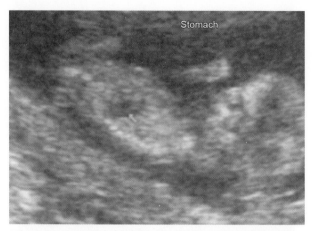

Fig. 4.51: Fetal stomach bubble seen in a fetus of 11 weeks and 4 days.

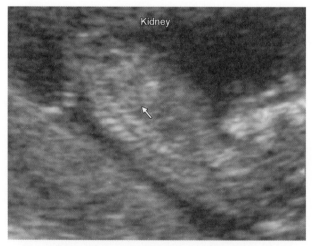

Fig. 4.52: Fetal kidney seen as an echogenic structure adjacent to the fetal spine.

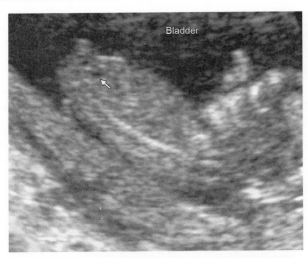

Fig. 4.53: Fetal urinary bladder seen in a fetus of 12 weeks and 2 days.

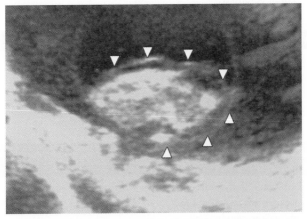

Fig. 4.54: Extensive cystic hygroma (arrowheads) in a 10 weeks and 1 day fetus.

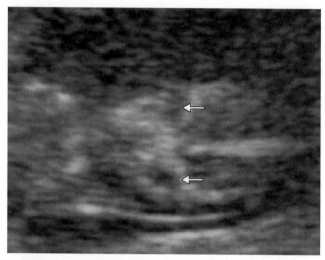

Fig. 4.55: Orbits (arrows) delineated as early as 11 weeks. Measure the ocular diameter, interocular distance and binocular distance to diagnose hypotelorism. Visualization of both orbits excludes anophthalmia or single orbit deformity.

TABLE 4.1: Ultrasound appearances of an early pregnancy failure.

- >5 mm embryo without cardiac activity (Fig. 4.56)
- >8 mm gestational sac without a yolk sac (Fig. 4.57)
- >16 mm gestational sac without an embryo (Fig. 4.58)
- Flaccid, large or irregular amniotic sac (Fig. 4.59)

TABLE 4.2: Ultrasound appearances of an impending early pregnancy failure.

- Embryonic bradycardia in relation with the gestational age
- Oligoamniotic sac (Fig. 4.60)
- Interval sac growth poor
- Abnormal shape or size of yolk sac (Figs. 4.61 and 4.62)

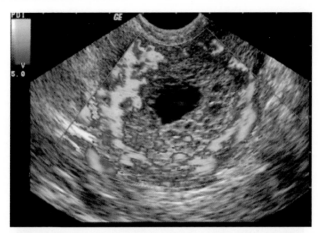

Fig. 4.56: Embryo 7 mm in size with no cardiac activity. Note the increase in peritrophoblastic vascularity which further helps in the diagnosis of an unhealthy pregnancy.

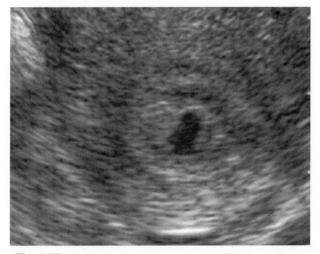

Fig. 4.57: Gestational sac, 12 mm in size without a yolk sac or a fetal node.

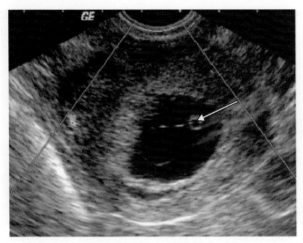

Fig. 4.58: Gestational sac, 26 mm in size with a yolk sac (arrow) but with no fetal node seen.

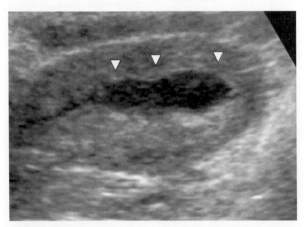

Fig. 4.59: Thin-walled, irregular and flaccid gestational sac of 7–8 weeks size with no yolk sac or embryo seen. Note the multiple foci of choriodecidual separation (arrowheads).

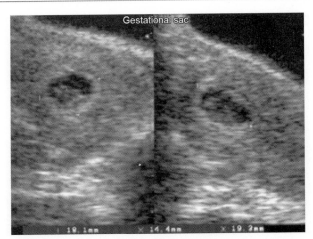

Fig. 4.60: Pregnancy of 7 weeks and 5 days showing an oligo-amniotic sac. The gestational sac size is 6 weeks and 2 days and the embryo size is 7 weeks and 4 days. The mean sac diameter is 17 mm and the crown rump length is 9 mm.

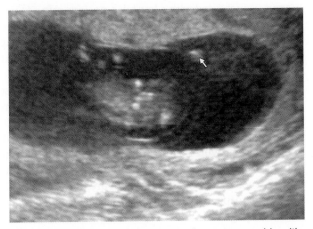

Fig. 4.61 : A hyperechoic shrunken yolk sac on one side with a cystic hygroma of the fetus seen as well.

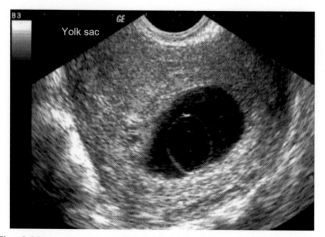

Fig. 4.62: Large yolk sec (15.6 mm) seen in the gestational sec

4.13 NUCHAL TRANSLUCENCY (TABLE 4.3)

- In 74–77 percent of trisomy 21 fetuses the fetal nuchal translucency is increased with a low false-positive rate.
- Sensitivity for detection of chromosomal abnormalities is extremely high by a combined screening of maternal age, fetal-nuchal translucency, nasal bone, ductus venosus and maternal biochemistry.
- The translucency (subcutaneous) between the skin and soft tissue posterior to the cervical spine has to be measured (Fig. 4.63).
- Nuchal translucency thickness usually increases with gestational age with 1.5 mm and 2.5 mm being the 50th and 95th percentile respectively for gestational ages between 10 and 12 weeks. 2.0 mm and 21.0 mm are the 50th and 95th percentile respectively for gestational ages between 12 and 14 weeks (Figs. 4.64 and 4.65).
- An increased nuchal translucency thickness (Figs. 4.66 to 4.70) not only indicates increased suspicion of

TABLE 4.3: Embryonic time table and its appearances on ultrasound.	
Structures visible on ultrasound	*No. of weeks from last menstrual period*
Gestational sac	4w4d–5w0d
Yolk sac	5w0d–5w3d
Embryonic pole	5w2d
Cardiac pulsations	5w3d
Limb buds	8w0d and >
Fetal movements	8w0d and >
Bowel herniation	9w0d–1 1w0d
Kidneys	10w0d and >
Choroid plexus	10w0d and >
Calcification of calvarium	10w0d and >
Orbits	10w4d and >
Stomach bubble	11w0d and>
Cardiac configuration	12w0d and >
Urinary bladder	12w0d and >

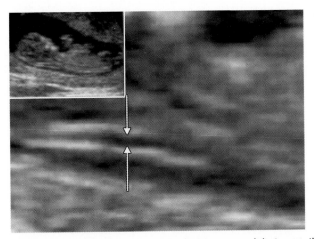

Fig. 4.63: The translucency (arrows) (subcutaneous) between the skin and soft tissue posterior to the cervical spine has to be measured.

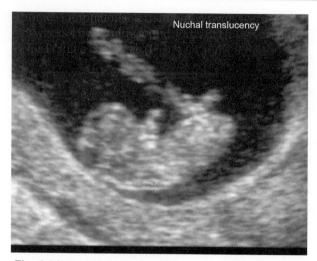

Fig. 4.64: Nuchal translucency thickness measurement in a
10 weeks size fetus.

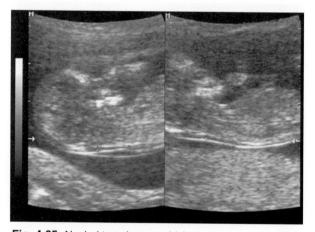

Fig. 4.65: Nuchal translucency thickness measurement in a
12 weeks size fetus.

chromosomal abnormalities but also indicates a possibility of multiple structural defects especially of the fetal heart and abdomen. Therefore, a normal karyotype does not in any way ensure normalcy of the fetus.

- A thickened nuchal translucency with spontaneous resolution and a normal nuchal skin fold thickness does not exclude a karyotypic abnormality.
- High risk patients for chromosomal abnormalities and cardiac defects should definitely be subjected to an ultrasound between 10 and 14 weeks for measurement of nuchal translucency thickness.

4.14 ABNORMAL FETUS

- Fetal abnormalities like Acrania (Fig. 4.71), Anencephaly (Fig. 4.72), Limb reduction defects, Gross anterior abdominal wall defects can be diagnosed in the late first trimester
  - Proboscis can be delineated on ultrasound as early as 12 weeks.

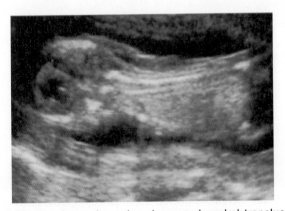

Fig. 4.66: The fetus showed an increased nuchal translucency thickness (0.5 mm at 12 weeks). An early amniocentesis showed a Trisomy 21 karyotype.

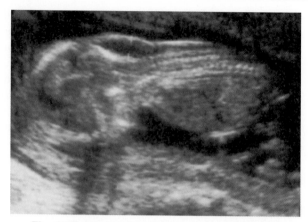

Fig. 4.67: Increased nuchal translucency thickness (6 mm at 13 weeks and 1 day).

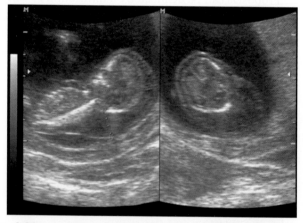

Fig. 4.68: Increased nuchal translucency thickness (5 mm at 12 weeks and 5 days). Patient refused an amniocentesis. Detailed anomaly scanning and fetal echocardiography at 18 weeks showed a transposition of great vessels.

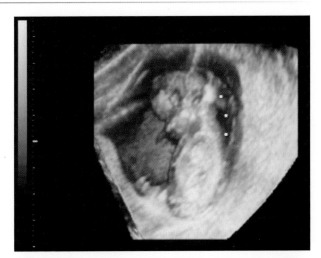

Fig. 4.69: Increased nuchal translucency as seen on 3D.

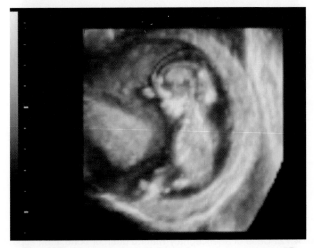

Fig. 4.70: Thickened nuchal translucency as seen on 3D.

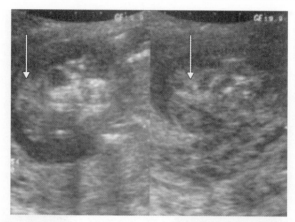

Fig. 4.71: Case of acrania with only brain and no bone seen superior to the orbits.

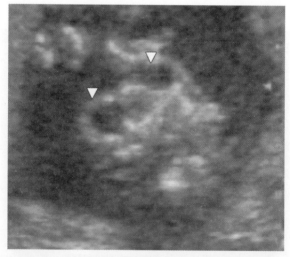

Fig. 4.72: Case of anencephaly with no brain or bone seen superior to the orbits.

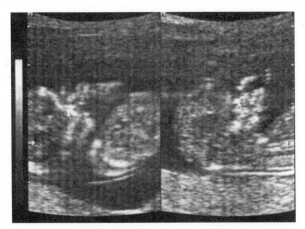

Fig. 4.73: Nasal bone ossification being present or absent is a marker for Trisomies especially Trisomy 21.

- Presence or absence of nasal bone along with nuchal translucency and ductus venosus flow velocity waveform are sensitive markers for chromosomal abnormali-ties.
  - Severe hypotelorism can also be delineated as orbits can be delineated from 11 weeks onwards
  - Single orbit, anophthalmia can also be diagnosed.
- Nasal bone ossification (Fig. 4.73) being absent can be diagnosed in the first trimester to raise the suspicion of chromosomal abnormalities.
- Thickened nuchal translucency can again raise the suspicion of chromosomal abnormalities and one can go in for early amniocentesis or biochemical markers to diagnose them. If nuchal translucency thickness resolves it does not indicate normalcy and on an amniocentesis if karyotype is normal subject the fetus to an echocardiography as an increased nuchal translucency thickness can denote a cardiac abnormality as well.

4.15 FIRST TRIMESTER SCAN CHECKLIST

- LMP and gestation
- Identify uterus and gestational sac do not hesitate to do a transvaginal scan
- Confirm viability and number
- Look at the cervix and implantation site
- Check adnexa
- Measure embryo
- Give a sonological gestational age and EDD and verify with LMP
- Give a complete structured report with hard copy of pictures.

4.16 DILEMMAS

- *Overdue:* Ultrasound or urine test. Urine test is positive before a gestational sac can be seen on an ultrasound scan.
- *Urine test negative:* Ultrasound to be done. Definitely to rule out any ectopic gestation and to confirm the cause for the delayed period.
- *Miscarried last time:* Should ultrasound be done. To be done to insure fetal well being and to discern any cause on ultrasound for recurrent pregnancy loss.
- *Pain in abdomen:* Ectopic will be definitely ruled out by ultrasound normally some or the other sign of ectopic pregnancy can be seen on an ultrasound scan, but many a times with overlapping nonspecific signs it can also be missed.

4.17 FIRST TRIMESTER KEY POINTS

- CRL = 10 mm= mean for 7 weeks
- CRL = 30 mm= mean for 9 weeks 5 days
- CRL = 60 mm= mean for 12 weeks 3 days
- A viable intrauterine pregnancy practically rules out ectopic gestation (Except one in 30000)

- There is a delay of identifying of one week by transabdominal as compared to transvaginal

Sac (2–4 mm)	4.5 weeks	5.5 weeks
Fetal heart (CRL 2–4)	5 weeks	6 weeks
Yolk sac (10 mm)	5 weeks	6 weeks

- Early fetal bradycardia signifies poor prognosis
- Fetal chromosomal anomalies can be screened for and detected in the 10–14 weeks scan
- Transvaginal scan does not increase abortion risk of bleeding
- A thorough knowledge of fetal embryology and implantation and corpus luteum physiology is a must for first trimester diagnosis.
- Do not hesitate to take second opinion
- 20 mm sac with no intrasac structures is suggestive of anembryonic pregnancy. A CRL of > 6 mm without fetal heart is suggestive of missed abortion. Confirm by TVS and repeat scan if required.

4.18 TRANSVAGINAL DECISION FLOWCHART

Failed pregnancy

4.19 DECISION-MAKING IN THE FIRST TRIMESTER

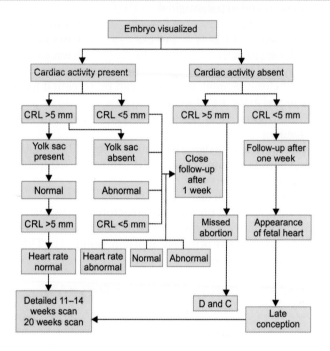

4.20 ULTRASOUND MARKERS OF CHROMOSOMAL ANOMALIES IN FIRST TRIMESTER

All pregnant women are at risk of carrying a fetus with genetic anomaly. Maternal age more than 35 years is no longer a criteria for screening as they carry only 30% of such pregnancies. The remaining occur in younger women making universal screening imperative. Advances in ultrasound machines and better training of professionals[1] have now made it possible to detect most of the chromosomal disorders in 11–13 weeks 6 days scan.

Advantages of early diagnosis being:
- Termination of pregnancy is safe and easy
- Privacy of the couple is maintained
- It is more accurate, far exceeding 2nd trimester triple test.
- Nuchal translucency—the most important criteria may regress after 14 weeks.
- Lesser bonding with the conceptus as compared to an advanced stage.
- If necessity arises CVS in experienced hands is as simple as amniocentesis.

Chromosomal anomalies are:
- Numerical
- Structural
- Single gene disorders.

Numerical anomalies are easily picked up by ultrasound alone and structural ones by ultrasound guided invasive procedures.

Incidence

As high as 50-60% in abortuses and app. 0.7% in new-borns. This difference is due to losses in 1st trimester, 2nd trimester, IUD and stillbirths.

The common aneuploidies are:
- Down syndrome (Trisomy 21)
- Edward's syndrome (Trisomy 18)
- Patau's syndrome (Trisomy 13)
- Turner's syndrome (Monosomy X)
- Triploidy
- Sex chromosome disorders.

Down syndrome is the most common chromosomal disorder (1 in 800 live births).[2] In 1866, Langdon Down reported that skin of 21 trisomy individual is too large than their body.[3] A century later Szabo and Gellen in 1990 described the association between Down syndrome and neck edema in the first trimester.[4]

What to look for at ultrasound for chromosomal anomalies

First and foremost is:

- Nuchal translucency (Fig. 4.74)
- Others being
- Nasal bone
- Frontomaxillary angle
- Ductus venosus flow velocity
- Tricuspid regurgitation
- Fetal heart rate.

Additional parameters may be:

- Maxillary length
- Ear length
- Flat iliac wings
- Megacystis
- Early onset IUGR.

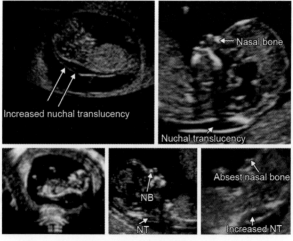

Fig. 4.74: Ultrasound for chromosomal anomalies: Nuchal translucency.

Nuchal translucency (NT)

This is the anechoic area at back of neck just adjacent to skin and bone and is formed by accumulation of fluid.[5] The term is translucency irrespective of thickness or septae. It usually resolves in 2nd trimester but may persist as cystic hygroma or nuchal edema.

Causes of increased NT are[6] cardiac failure, superior mediastinal compression causing venous congestion, altered composition of extracellular matrix, abnormal or delayed development of lymphatic system, abnormal fetal lymphatic drainage due to diminished fetal movements and fetal anemia.

Consequently anomalies can be:
- Chromosomal
- Cardiac defects
- Pulmonary malformations
- Skeletal dysplasias
- Intrauterine infections
- Metabolic disorders
- Hematological disorders.

How to Measure
- True sagittal section
- CRL between 45–85 mm (11–13.6 weeks)
- Only head and upper third of thorax on screen
- Neutral position of fetal neck
- Amnion not to be included
- To exclude umbilical cord near neck. Color Doppler may be very useful[7]
- Spine should be at bottom of image
- Calipers to be placed next to lucent area which should not be included
- 3D ultrasound increases the accuracy of measurement.[8]

Normal values

- Range from 1.2 to 2.1 mm at 45 mm CRL and up to 1.9 to 2.7 mm at 85 mm CRL.
- Few normal fetuses may also have increased NT.

Fetal Nasal Bone (FNB) is gaining popularity in past few years. FNB is absent or hypoplastic in 69% of trisomy 21, 50% of trisomy 18 and 30% of trisomy 13 and 1.4% of chromosomally normal fetuses in 11 to 13 weeks 6 days scan. It may appear in these cases with increase in gestational age (Fig. 4.75).

It is assessed in same section as NT. Transducer should be parallel to direction of nose.

Fetal facial angle or frontomaxillary facial angle (FMP angle) This angle becomes wider in such fetuses due to small maxilla. It decreases with increasing CRL. It is also measured in the same image as NT and NB. Angle is measured between

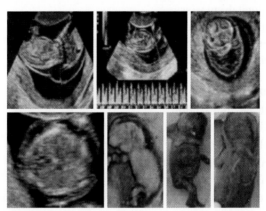

Fig. 4.75: Trisomy 13 and increased nuchal translucency at 12th weeks of gestation. Sagittal section by 2D ultrasound shows increased NT. Fetal ductus venosus shows reverse a wave. Transverse section of head also shows nuchal edema. Surface rendered image of the fetus by 3D u/s. Post abortive pictures of the fetus shows fluid filled structures around the neck (left to right respectively). Fetal Karyotyping by CVS revealed trisomy 13.

a line along the superior surface of the palate and a line drawn from the anteriosuperior corner of the maxilla to the anterior surface of frontal bones. When CRL is 45 mm facial angle is 83 degrees decreasing to 75 at CRL of 84 mm.

Ductus venosus: It is an independent marker. 80.5% of trisomy 21 while 5% of normal fetuses show decrease or reversal of flow in ductus venosus in 11–13 weeks 6 days scan, used only at tertiary centers. It is a useful complementary method for reducing invasive testing rate and increasing reassurance from a negative result.

Tricuspid regurgitation(TR): If seen increases the risk of trisomy 21 as well as cardiac defects. TR is diagnosed if found during at least half of the duration of the systole with a velocity of greater than 60 cm/sec. Fetuses with TR and normal karyotype should be assessed for cardiac defects.

Other parameters: Fifty percent of fetuses with trisomy 21 have a maxillary length 0. 7 mm less than the normal median for CRL. A short ear length, femur and humerus are not of much significance at this gestational age.

A single umbilical artery shows a seven fold increase in risk of trisomy 18.

An abnormally large urinary bladder (megacystis) if present increases the likelihood of trisomy13 and 18 by a factor of 6.7. If fetus is chromosomally normal it resolves in 90% cases spontaneously. Incidence of chromosomal anomalies is app.10% if bladder is more than 15 mm.

Combined with modern biochemical markers the detection rate increases thus reducing invasive procedures markedly.

CONCLUSION

A pregnancy should never be terminated on these findings alone. In fetuses with abnormal NT and normal karyotype, risk of other congenital anomalies is higher, and hence detailed anomaly scan at 19 weeks should be advised.

REFERENCES

1. Mahieu-Caputo D, Senat MV, Romana S, et al. What's new in fetal medicine? Arch Pediatr. 2002;22:296-307.
2. Thompson M, McInnes R, Willard H. Thompson and Thompson Genetics in Medicine. 5th ed. Philadelphia, Pa:WB Saunders; 1991.
3. Langdon Down J. Observations on an ethnic classification of idiots. Clin Lectures and Reports, London Hospital. 1866;3:259-62.
4. Szabo J, Gellen J. Nuchal fluid accumulation in trisomy-21 detected by vaginal sonography in first trimester. Lancet. 1990;336:1133.
5. Nicolaides KH, Azar G, Byrne D, et al. Fetal nuchal translucency: ultrasound screening for chromosomal defects in first trimester of pregnancy. Br Med J. 1992;304:867-9.
6. Nicolaides KH , Sebire NJ, Snijders RJM. Pathophysiology of increased nuchal translucency. In the 11-14 weeks scan: the diagnosis of fetal abnormalities. Carnforth, UK: Patherson Publishing, 1999;95-13 .
7. Schafer M, Laurichesse-Delmas H, Ville Y. The effect of nuchal cord on nuchal translucency measurement at 10–14 weeks. Ultrasound Obstet Gynecol. 1998;11:271.
8. Wee LK, Chai HY, Supriyanto E. Surface Rendering of Three dimensional ultrasound images using VTK. J. Sci. Indust. Res, 2011;70(6):421-6.

4.21 FIRST TRIMESTER BIOCHEMICAL MARKERS AND NONINVASIVE SCREENING

Universal screening is a strategy applied to all individuals of a certain category to identify a high risk group to have an unrecognized disease in individuals without signs or symptoms of such disease. A test used in a screening program, especially for a disease with low incidence, must have a high detection rate and low false positive rate. In screening by maternal age with a cut off age 38 years, 5% of population is high risk having 30% of Down's babies.[1]

Over the past 35 years there has been a steady evolution of biophysical as well as biochemical parameters used to know the risk that a woman is carrying a fetus with aneuploidy.

First Trimester Biochemical Markers

Biochemical Markers in 1st trimester are:

- Free beta hCG[2]
- Pregnancy associated plasma protein (PAPP-A)[2] and very recent ones
- Pregnancy-specific beta-1 glycoprotein (SP1)-Time window 7–12 weeks
- ADAM-12 (A disintegrin and metalloprotease). It is more pronounced earlier in pregnancy and is reduced in Down's syndrome (Liagaard et al. 2006).

Week	8–9	10–11	12–13
ADAM-12 (MoMs)	0.12	0.50	0.93

Markers profile of a pregnancy with DS in first trimester

NT	High
Free β-hCG	High (2.0 × normal)
PAPP-A	Low (0.4 × normal)
ADAM-12	Low (as depicted above)

CHEMICAL MARKERS WITH CHROMOSOME ABNORMALITIES

	β-hCG	PAPP-A
T21	↑	↓
T18	↓	↓
T13	↓	↓
Triploidy (paternal)	↑↑↑	↓
Triploidy (maternal)	↓↓	↓↓
Sex chromosome abnormalities	→	↓

In normal euploid pregnancies the average free β-hCG is 1.0 MoM and PAPP-A is 1.0 MoM.

First trimester screening for trisomies 21, 18, and 13 by a combination of maternal age, fetal nuchal translucency thickness (NT), fetal heart rate (FHR), and serum free beta human chorionic gonadotropin (fbhCG) and pregnancy-associated plasma protein-A {PAPP-A) can detect about 90% of cases of trisomy 21 and 95% of those with trisomies 18 and 13, at FPR of about 5%. The performance of first trimester screening can be improved by expanding the combined test to include nasal bone, ductus venosus, pulsatility index and tricuspid regurgitation.

There are different protocols for screening of chromosomal defects.

- **Combined test** in 1st trimester
- **Sequential tests** in 1st and 2nd trimester
    - *Integrated* not telling the results of 1st trimester till 2nd trimester results are available
    - *Stepwise sequential:* 1st trimester NT + PAPP-A + fb-hCG. Those with low risk (higher cut off) get 2nd trimester AFP, uE3, fb-hCG and inhibin, and the risk is calculated from all 7 markers.
    - *Contingent test:* It is more efficient. 1st trimester NT+PAPP-A+ fb-hCG. Women with very high risk are offered invasive prenatal diagnosis and only those with borderline risk are offered 2nd trimester AFP, uE3, fb-hCG and inhibin. Their risk is estimated from all 7 markers. This group has such a low risk that it is unlikely that further markers will lead to a final high risk result.

Method of screening[3]	Detection rate
Maternal age (MA)	30
MA and fetal nuchal translucency (NT) at 11–13 + 6 weeks	70-8
MA and NT and maternal serum free β-hCG and PAPP-A at 11–13 + 6 weeks	85-9
MA and NT and fetal nasal bone (NB) at 11–13 + 6 weeks	90
MA and fetal NT and NB and maternal serum free β-hCG and PAPP-A at 11–13 + 6 weeks (The last is a sort of contingent screening in 1st trimester)	95

Noninvasive Prenatal Diagnosis and Testing

This test is based on the analysis of extracellular deoxyribonucleic acid (DNA) measured in the blood of pregnant women; cell free fetal DNA (cffDNA) (Fig. 4.76). Small fragments of fetal DNA circulate freely in maternal blood.[4] Cell free fetal DNA was first discovered by Lo et al in 1997. Fetal DNA comes from the placenta. Cff DNA is mixed with a larger proportion of maternal cell free DNA. The first application of this phenomenon focused on the detection, or exclusion of, paternally-inherited fetal DNA sequences that are not present in mother such as Y chromosome sequences in pregnancies with a male fetus or rhesus D sequences in women who are Rh –ve. Recently DNA technologies have allowed precise relative quantification of DNA fragments and now it can be done in a robust manner.

On average they represent 10% of total circulating DNA. The life cycle of these cells is of less than 2 hours.[5] and are not found after birth. As in cases of fetal trisomy, there are three copies instead of two, there is increase in their presence.

This test can be undertaken from as early as 10th week. of pregnancy with results available in a week. It can detect 99% cases of trisomy 21, 97% of trisomy 18 and 92% of trisomy 13 with respective FPR's of 0.08%, 0.15% and 0.2%. The main limitation is the test failure rate of up to 4% due to lesser concentration of fetal part. This is higher as body mass index of mother increases; the test failure rate is 50% at maternal weight of 160 kg.

The International Federation of Gynecology and Obstetrics (FIGO) recommends the following:

- Maternal age has low performance as a screening for fetal chromosomal abnormalities with a DR of 30–50% for FPR of 5–20%. Therefore, invasive *testing for diagnosis of fetal aneuploidies should not be carried out by taking into account only maternal age.*

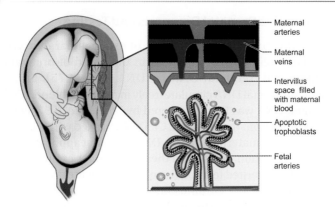

Fig. 4.76: Cell free fetal DNA shedding into maternal bloodstream.

- First line screening for trisomies 21, 18 and 13 should be achieved by the combined test, which takes into account maternal age, fetal nuchal translucency (NT) thickness, fetal heart rate (FHR) and maternal serum free β-hCG and PAPP-A. The combined test has a DR of 90% for trisomy 21 and 95% for trisomies 18 and 13, at FPR of about 5%.

- The combined test could be improved by assessing additional ultrasonographic markers, including the fetal nasal bone and Doppler assessment of the fetal ductus venosus flow and tricuspid flow. If all these markers are included the DR is increased to more than 95% and the FPR decreased to less than 3%.

- Screening by analysis of cfDNA in maternal blood has a DR of 99% for trisomy 21, 97% for trisomy 18 and 92% for trisomy 13, at a total FPR of 0.4%.

- Clinical implementation of cfDNA testing should preferably be in a contingent strategy, based on the results of first-line screening by the combined test at 11–13 weeks. In this case, we recommend the strategy below:

 – Combined test risk over **1 in 100:** The patients can be offered the options of cfDNA testing or invasive testing.
 – Combined test risk between **1 in 101 and 1 in 2500:** patients can be offered the option of cfDNA testing.
 – Combined test risk lower than **1 in 2500:** There is no need for further testing.

Patients contemplating pregnancy termination following a positive result from cfDNA testing should be advised that the diagnosis should be confirmed by invasive testing before undertaking any further action.

REFERENCES

1. Snijders RJM, Sundberg K, Holzgreve W, et al. Maternal age and gestation specific risk for trisomy 21. Ultrasound Obstet Gynecol. 1999;13:167-70.
2. Krantz DA, Larsen JW, Buchanan PD, et al. First trimester Down syndrome screening: free beta-human chorionic gonadotropin and pregnancy-associated plasma protein A. Am J Obstet zynecol. 1996;174:612-6.
3. WWW.Fetal medicine foundation.
4. Lo YM, Chamberlain PF, Rai V, et al. Presence of fetal DNA in maternal plasma and serum. Lancet. 1997;350:485-7 [Pub Med].
5. Lo YM, Zhang J, Leung TN, et al. Rapid clearance of fetal DNA from maternal plasma. Am J Hum Genet. 1999;64:218-24.

4.22. FIRST TRIMESTER: DETECTION OF NON-CHROMOSOMAL ANOMALIES

11–13 weeks scan has evolved over the last 25 years from essentially a scan for measurement of fetal NT and CRL to one which includes a basic checklist for examination of fetal anatomy with the intention of diagnosing major abnormalities, which are either lethal or are associated with severe handicap, so that the parents can have the option of earlier and safer termination of pregnancy.

INTRODUCTION

First Trimester Diagnosis:
- Possible with transvaginal ultrasound
- Best opportunity: 11 to 14 weeks scan

Ongoing definition continue for:
- Some malformations
- Timeline for visualization
- Effectiveness

The detection of fetal anomalies in the first trimester is made possible with the advent of high frequency transvaginal probes, which has resulted in defining a number of malformations and clarifying the optimal gestational age to visualize anatomical structures. Systematic screening during the late first trimester (11 to 14 weeks scan) yields the greatest opportunity to define certain abnormalities, while there remains a need to evaluate and further define the effectiveness and place for early fetal assessment.[1]

METHODS

Select transverse section of head to demonstrate skull, midline echo and choroid plexuses; a mid sagittal view of face to demonstrate nasal bone; sagittal section of the spine for kyphoscoliosis; a transverse section of the thorax for four chamber view of heart and record blood flow across the tricuspid valve; and transverse and sagittal section of the trunk and extremities to demonstrate the stomach, bladder, abdominal insertion of the umbilical cord, all the long bones, hands and feet.

Overall First Trimester Detection

First Trimester Diagnosis of Malformations:
- 50% detection at 11 to 14 weeks
- 93% detection in combination with mid-trimester scan
- 33% complete normal anatomy seen
- 50% average detection sensitivity (systematic review)

Unable to define all malformations due to:
- Late organ development
- Developmental sequence of malformations

In a prospective study of 1148 singleton pregnancies at 11 to 14 weeks, 50% of major structural malformations, were detected, while a 2-stage process with a second mid-trimester scan detected 42.8% of more abnormalities for a total detection rate of 92.8%.[2] Complete fetal anatomy was seen in 33% of cases at 11 to 13 6/7 weeks in 1 study, while the cranium, intracranial anatomy, face, cord insertion, stomach and 4 limbs were seen in 95% of cases and fetal heart in 84%. In a systematic review encompassing 19 studies, the average sensitivity for first trimester detection of abnormalities was 50%.[3] In the future, 3-dimensional virtual reality ultrasound may increase the first trimester detection rate for certain malformations such as those of the skeleton and skin. Due to the late development of some organs as well as the developmental sequence of malformations, first trimester ultrasound will not be able to detect all defects.

Nuchal Translucency and Non-chromosomal Abnormalities

NT is a fluid filled subcutaneous space in the posterior neck region that can be reliably measured from 10 weeks 3 days to 13 weeks 6 days gestational age.

Nuchal Translucency and Adverse Pregnancy Outcomes

NT and Adverse Pregnancy Outcome:
- *Adverse outcomes:* Fetal malformations, dysplasia deformations, disruptions and genetic syndromes
- Significant when NT ≥3.5 mm (>99th percentile)
- *No increased risk with:* Survival to mid-trimester plus no abnormalities on targeted scan.

In addition to its strong association with fetal aneuploidies, increased NT is linked to the risk of adverse perinatal outcomes including fetal malformations, dysplasias, deformations, disruptions and genetic syndromes, but these risks do not reach significance until the NT is ≥3.5 mm (>99th percentile).[4] The fetal death rate depends upon the degree of abnormality of the NT (at 3.5–4.4 mm, death rate = 2.7%, at >6.5 mm, death rate = 19%). Alternatively, if the fetus survives to the mid-trimester and no abnormalities are noted on the targeted scan, the risk of adverse outcome does not significantly increase.

Specialized training and certification for sonographers is required for the NT measurement. A calculator is available on *Perinatology.com*. If the CRL is known, the estimated gestational age and expected nuchal translucency can be obtained. If the NT measurement is known, the calculator will yield the NT percentile.

First Trimester Non-chromosomal Abnormalities

The first-trimester examination offers additional benefits for confirming gestational age and viability, identifying other structural malformations, and suggesting potential pregnancy complications stillbirths, preterm delivery, preeclampsia, gestational diabetes, and fetal macrosomia).

Non-chromosomal Anomalies: 11–14 week scan
Some structural noncardiac anomalies detected: • *CNS:* Acrania, alobar holoprosencephaly, exomphalos anencephaly, exencephaly   • *Abdomen or related:* Gastroschisis, omphalocele megacystis, and body stalk   • *Others:* 50% diaphragmatic hernia and 50% lethal skeletal dysplasia   • *Difficult to detect:* Agenesis of corpus callosum.

In fetuses without chromosomal anomalies, certain malformations are commonly detected at the 11–14 week scan, especially those of the CNS (acrania, alobar holo-prosencephaly, and exomphalos) and of the abdomen (gastroschisis, megacystis, and body stalk anomaly), while others are less commonly defined (50% diaphragmatic hernia and 50% lethal skeletal dysplasias).[5] In the same study, non-detected malformations included agenesis of the corpus callosum, cerebellar hypoplasia, echogenic lung lesions, bowel obstruction and renal defects.

Nuchal Translucency and Congenital Heart

Nuchal Translucency (NT) and Congenital Heart Disease:
- NT >95th percentile: present in about one-third of fetuses with major cardiac defects
- Risk is dependent upon degree of NT abnormality
- If NT ≥ 3.5 mm, heart defects: 1 in 43 singleton pregnancies.

Disease

In fetuses without chromosomal abnormalities, the incidence of congenital heart disease is increased in those with an NT value above the 95th percentile, which is present in approximately one-third of fetuses with major cardiac defects. The risk is dependent upon the degree of NT abnormality and when the NT is ≥3.5 mm, heart defects are present in 1 of 43 singleton pregnancies.[6]

NT and Congenital Heart Disease (CHD):
- *NT >95th percentile:* Present in about one-third of fetuses with major cardiac defects
- *Risk of CHD:* Dependent upon degree of NT abnormality
- If NT is ≥ 3.5 mm, CHD incidence is 6.0% (5.2–6.8%),
- If NT is 3.5 to 4.4 mm, CHD incidence is 3.2% (2.3–4.1%),
- If NT is >4.5 mm, CHD incidence is 11.8% (9.8 to 13.8%).
(See below GoetzJ review)

Goetzl has reviewed the literature on this topic and when the NT is ≥3.5 mm, the incidence of overall cardiac

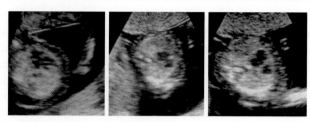

Fig. 4.77: Transverse section of the fetal chests in the fetuses with increased NT at first trimester. A VSD, single ventricle and dextraposition of fetal heart are seen.

abnormalities is 6.0% (5.2–6.8%); when the NT is 3.5 to 4.4 mm, the incidence is 3.2% (2.3–4.1 %); and when the NT is >4.5 mm, the incidence is 11.8% (9.8–13.8%) (Fig. 4.77).

CHD in High Risk

CHD First Trimester High Risk Groups
Risk groups:
Increased NT
Tricuspid regurgitation (TR)
Reversal or absence of "a" wave in Ductus Venosus (Abnormal DV)
If NT >99th percentile or abnormal DV/Detection rate for CHD = 47% with false positive 2.7%
TR + increased NT + abnormal DV flow → 78% Sensitivity for CHD detection.

Groups

A combination of increased NT and the observations of tricuspid regurgitation as well as reversal of the "a" wave in the ductus venosus is predictive of major cardiac defects.[7] When the NT is above the 99th percentile or the ductus venosus A-wave is absent or reversed, a 47% detection rate for major cardiac defects is reported with a 2.7% false positive rate.

Tricuspid regurgitation (TR) observed in the first trimester is present in approximately 7% of normal fetuses and has a significant association with fetal aneuploidy, especially in the presence of other markers but as an isolated finding, TR demonstrates a low screening potential for fetal aneuploidy and congenital heart defects.

With qualified personnel and equipment, detection of major CHD in high-risk groups (TR, increased NT, abnormal DV flow) is reported with a sensitivity of 78.5% in the first and early second trimester.

First Trimester Diagnosis CHD:
Early diagnosis CHD requires: Caution, high level of expertise and equipment, and knowledge of potentially high false positive rates.

Finally, fetal echocardiography in the first trimester has limitations and assessment of the fetal heart at this gestational requires a high level of expertise and caution is advised. In one review, the false positive rate is reported as high as 33%, while in expert hands the false positive rate is much lower.

Central Nervous System (CNS) Malformations

First Trimester CNS Malformations

Detectable major CNS malformations:
- Acrania anencephaly sequence
- Holoprosencephaly
- Cerebellar defects
- Hydranencephaly
- Encephalocele
- Spina bifida
- Specialized views may enable diagnosis of posterior fossa abnormalities.

A number of structural CNS malformations are seen during the first trimester and include:[8] acrania anencephaly sequence, holoprosencephaly, cerebellar defects, hydranencephaly,

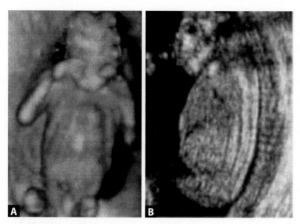

Figs. 4.78A and B: Acrania at 1st trimester. 3D surface rendered image (A) and 2D sagittal section (B) of the body and extremities.

encephalocele and spina bifida (Figs. 4.78 to 4.80). Enlargement of intracranial translucency and enlargement of the brainstem to occipital bone are potential markers for posterior fossa abnormalities during the first trimester. Sonographers can be trained to perform intracranial translucency measurements at the 11 to 13 week examination, resulting in reproducible results. In the detection of spina bifida in the first trimester, the non-visualization of the posterior fossa (cisterna magna) is reported as the best screening method.

Kidneys

Renal Malformations:
- *First trimester:* Bladder normally seen 90% of cases
- *Megacystis:* 38% of cases detected

During the first trimester, the bladder is normally visualized in about 90% of cases. Among fetuses with megacystis,

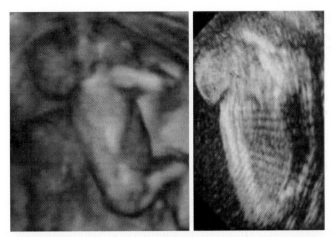

Fig. 4.79: Encephalocele at 13 weeks. 3D and 2D images clearly show the abnormality.

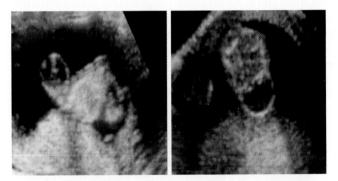

Fig. 4.80: 2D Ultrasound sagittal and transverse sections show anencephaly at 10 weeks.

about 38% were detected during the first trimester and the main etiologies were urethral occlusion and prune-belly syndrome, both of which carry a poor prognosis.[9]

Abdomen

First Trimester Abdomen and Other Abnormalities

Malformations detected:

Anterior abdominal wall defects:

- Body stalk anomaly (fetal body attached to placenta, spine angulation)
- Omphalocele (bowel herniation after 12 weeks)
- Gastroschisis (bowel herniates into amniotic cavity, cord inserts laterally) (Figs. 4.81A to C)

Other abnormalities detected:

- Cleft lip
- Diaphragmatic hernia
- Skeletal dysplasia

Among abdominal defects, anterior abdominal wall defects are possible to detect during the first trimester (Figs. 4.81A to C). Body stalk abnormality is characterized by a malformed fetus with an anterior abdominal wall defect and a portion of the fetal body attached to the placenta, while a key finding is angulation of the fetal spine and kyphoscoliosis. Omphalocele occurs when there is herniation of the fetal bowel beyond 12 weeks gestation with cord insertion at the apex of the herniated sac. Gastroschisis is an anterior abdominal wall defect in which bowel herniates into the amniotic cavity with the cord insertion lateral to the defect.

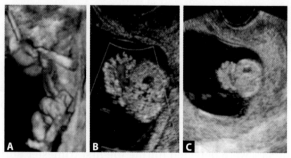

Figs. 4.81A to C: Gastroschisis at 1st trimester 3D surface rendered image clearly shows fetal intestines protruding from the anterior abdominal wall defect (A) on the left. 2D U/S (C) and color flow of transverse section (B).

Other Abnormalities

Other potential abnormalities seen in the first trimester are: Cleft lip, diaphragmatic hernia with stomach visualized in the chest and mediastinal shift, and skeletal dysplasia with abnormal long bones, contractures and altered echogenicity.[10]

REFERENCES

1. Timor-Tritsch IEl, Fuchs KM, Monteagudo A, et al. Performing a fetal anatomy scan at the time of first-trimester screening. Obstet Gynecol. 2009;13(2 Pt 1):402-7.

2. Souka APl, Pilalis A, Kavalakis I, et al. Screening for major structural abnormalities at the 11- to 14-week ultrasound scan. Am J Obstet Gynecol. 2006;194(2):393-6.

3. Farraposo S, Montenegro N, Matias A. Evaluation of the role of first-trimester obstetric ultrasound in the detection of major anomalies: a systematic review. J Perinat Med. 2014;42(2):141-9.

4. Souka APl, Von Kaisenberg CS, Hyett JA, et al. Increased nuchal translucency with normal karyotype. Am J Obstet Gynecol. 2005; 192(4): 1005-21.

5. Syngelaki A 1, Chelemen T, Dagklis T, et al. Challenges in the diagnosis of fetal non-chromosomal abnormalities at 11-13 weeks. Prenat Diagn. 2011;31(1):90-102.

6. Bahado-Singh ROI, Wapner R, Thom E, et al. First Trimester Maternal Serum Biochemistry and Fetal Nuchal Translucency Screening Study Group. Elevated first-trimester nuchal translucency increases the risk of congenital heart defects. Am J Obstet Gynecol. 2005;192 (5):1357-61.

7. Mogra Rl, Alabbad N, Hyett J. Increased nuchal translucency and congenital heart disease. Early Hum Dev. 2012;88(5):261-7.

8. Goetz! L. Adverse pregnancy outcomes after abnormal first-trimester screening for aneuploidy. Clin Lab Med. 2010;30(3): 613-28.

9. Fievet L, Faure A, Coze S, et al. Fetal megacystis: etiologies, management, and outcome according to the trimester. Urology. 2014;84(1):185-90.

10. Goetzl L. Adverse pregnancy outcomes after abnormal first-trimester screening for aneuploidy. Clin Lab Med. 2010;30(3):613-28.

4.23 THREE DIMENSIONAL SONOEMBRYOLOGY

3D sonography has established itself in recent years due to development of computer processor technology. Modern 3D systems are capable to generate surface and transparent views depicting the sculpture like reconstruction of fetal surface structures and X-ray like images of fetal skeleton. Image quality is extremely important to delineate the origin and extension of a congenital anomaly. Clear images and elimination of redundant structures and artifacts allows better understanding of fetal structures.

There is an increasing body of research which indicates that 3D images may improve the accuracy of anomaly detection of the fetal face, ears, and distal extremities when compared to 2D images (Figs. 4.82 and 4.83).

3D technique is complementary, not alternative to 2D technique in the field of prenatal diagnosis.[1] 3D provides a diagnostic gain in many cases.

It has 2 modes—Planar and full three dimensional.

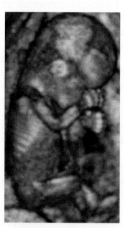

Fig. 4.82: 3D image of a fetus in the late first trimester.

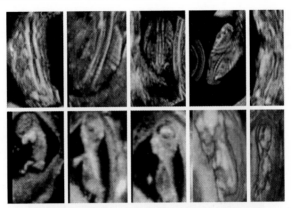

Fig. 4.83: Fetal spine can be evaluated successfully at the first trimester by 2D (above line) and 3D ultrasound VCI technique (bottom first 3 pictures) and 3D surface rendered image(last 2 on the right at the bottom line).

Planar mode: The object is simultaneously projected to three perpendicular planes. There is no limit to object rotation and number of tomograms.

Full three dimensional mode: It is particularly useful in presenting three dimensional interrelationship of different organs or skeleton. Sonographer can optionally change different modalities of image rendering emphasizing the outer surface or presenting inner structures through the transparent mode.

Limitations

- Long learning curve
- Fetal and maternal movements during scanning can lead to motion artifacts that can degrade quality of image.[2,3]

Advantages

- 3D is particularly useful in study of nuchal translucency (100% v/s 85% by 2D)
- Ectopics, planar mode can distinguish true and pseudo-gestational sacs.

- Thoraco-omphalopagus conjoined twins were diagnosed at 9 weeks 4 by 3D ultrasound. Early diagnosis of conjoined twins is still a challenge (Figs. 4.84 and 4.85).

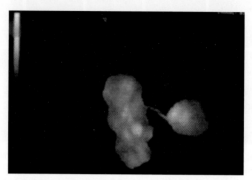

Fig. 4.84: 3D TVS image of 7–8 weeks gestation by surface mode, Note regular shape of yolk sac.

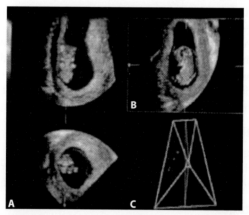

Figs. 4.85A to C: 3D scan of a 12 Weeks. fetus. Plane (A) allows a frontal view of fetal nuchal region; Plane (B) shows an ideal Sagittal view of the fetus; Plane (C) gives a symmetrical transverse section of the fetus. These planes make measurement of nuchal translucency much easier and more accurate.

- Yolk sac volume can be accurately measured and thus outcome of pregnancy predicted (Fig. 4.84).[5]

CONCLUSION

The latest achievement in the field of 3D/4D Ultrasound is the high definition live (HD live) technology. The virtual light source produces selective illumination. Virtual light can be placed in the front, back or lateral sides until a clear image is achieved.

REFERENCES

1. Mirik-Tesanic D, Kurjak A. Trodimenzionalni ultrazvuk u ginekoiogiji I porodnistvu. Ginekol Perinatol. 1997;6:43-46.
2. Baba K, Satch K, Sakamoto S, et al. Development of an ultrasonic system for three-dimensional reconstruction of the fetus. J Perinat Med. 1989;17:19-24.
3. Pretorius DH, Nelson TR. Three-dimensional ultrasound. Opininon. Ultrasound Obstet Gynecol. 1995;5:219-21.
4. Meizner I, Levy A, Katz M, et al. Early ultrasonic diagnosis of conjoined twins. Harefuah. 1993;124:741-4,196.
5. Lindsay DJ, Lyons EA, Levi CS, et al. Endovaginal appearance of the yolk sac in early pregnancy: normal growth and usefulness as a predictor of abnormal pregnancy outcome. Radiology. 1988;166:109-12.

4.24 COLOR DOPPLER IN FIRST TRIMESTER

The data available till date suggest that diagnostic ultrasound has no adverse effects on embryogenesis or fetal growth. However, the safety of color, pulsed and power Doppler remains a concern. They should be performed with caution due to possible thermal effects.[1,2] In particular use of pulsed Doppler involves use of higher intensities compared to diagnostic ultrasound, and hence may cause significant heating and thermal effects. Risk can be minimized by limiting dwell time, limiting exposure to critical structures and following equipment generated exposure information. When performing

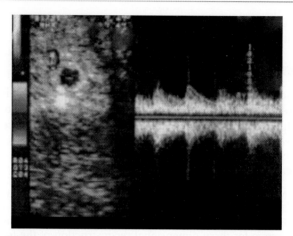

Fig. 4.86: Transvaginal color Doppler image of an early gestational sac. Blood flow signals derived from spiral arteries demonstrate low vascular resistance (PI = 0.77).

Doppler imaging the thermal index (T1) should be <1.0 and exposure short, no longer than 5–10 min (Fig. 4.86).

INDICATIONS

Diagnosing Early Gestation Sac

Earliest sonographic features of uterine pregnancy is demonstration of a focal echogenic area of thickening in endometrial stripe—intradecidual sign. By color Doppler we can see tiny spiral arteries coming up to the sac.

ASSESSING VIABILITY OF EARLY PREGNANCY USING TRANSVAGINAL COLOR DOPPLER (FIG. 4.86)

It has been helpful in distinguishing between normal and a failed pregnancy. High velocity peritrophoblastic flow with low impedance is suggestive of normal intrauterine gestation sac.

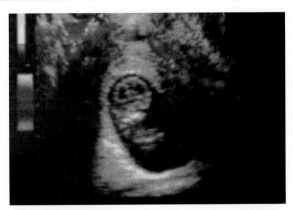

Fig. 4.87: Transvaginal color Doppler scan of a missed abortion. Prominent blood flow signals are obtained from spiral arteries while absence of heart activity is noted by color Doppler.

Intradecidual flow with PSV > 15 cm/sec is suggestive of intrauterine gestation sac even before gestation sac is seen.[3] RI < 0.55

Inadequate trophoblastic invasion of the spiral arteries and Rl >0.55 in decidual spiral arteries is indicative of increased incidence of pregnancy failure (Fig. 4.87).

Absence of heart beats and the lack of color flow signals at its expected position in fetus after the 6th gestational week suggests fetal demise.

Pulsatility index (PI) is higher in patients with recurrent pregnancy loss, PI > 3.08 ± 0.61 at 4–5 weeks of gestation.

PERIGESTATIONAL HEMORRHAGE

Ectopic Pregnancy

Color Doppler can differentiate between pseudogestational sac of ectopic pregnancy and gestational sac of intrauterine pregnancy. Pseudogestational sac is characterized by either absent flow around it or very low velocity flow (<8 cm/s peak systolic velocity) and moderate resistance to flow (RI > 0.50).[4] Normal or abnormal intrauterine gestational sac has high velocity and low resistance pattern (RI < 0.45).[5]

Randomly dispersed multiple small vessels are seen in the adnexa showing high velocity and low impedance signals (RI = 0.36–0.45) clearly separated from the ovarian tissue and corpus luteum (Fig. 4.88).

Leash sign–All cases of tubal ectopic have a typical eccentric leash of vessels on color Doppler that shows a low resistance placental type of flow on spectral Doppler. This sign has a sensitivity of 100% and specificity of 99%, a positive predictive value of 95% and negative predictive value of 100% thus helping in the diagnosis of ectopic pregnancy early, resulting in decreased morbidity and mortality.[6]

If no gestational sac is seen in adnexa, color Doppler can differentiate ectopic and corpus luteum.

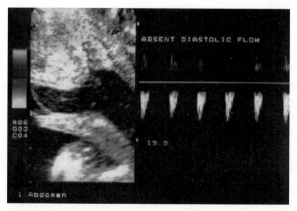

Fig. 4.88: Transvaginal color Doppler scan of a hematoma. Note the absence of diastolic flow (RI = 1.0) detected in spiral arteries close to perigestational hemorrhage.

In a study RI for ectopic was 0.36 ± 0.02 SD, whereas it was 0.48 ± 0.04 SD for corpora lutea. A cut-off value of 0.40 or less is proposed as a diagnostic index of trophoblast in adnexa.

Visualization of ipsilateral corpus luteum blood flow may aid in the diagnosis of ectopic pregnancy.

RETAINED PRODUCTS OF CONCEPTION

Thick endometrium with inhomogenus contents within, showing focal increased vascularity-low resistance flow (RI < 0.45) going into myometrium or just beneath the endometrial-myometrial interface (Fig. 4.89).

OVARIAN MASSES

Corpus luteal cyst-usually < 5 cm in size with clear contents, sometimes larger in size and may show internal echoes–suggestive of internal hemorrhage.

Usually regresses in size in follow-up scans.

Power Doppler study shows Ring of fire vascularity.

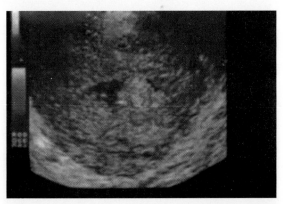

Fig. 4.89: TVS Power Doppler image of an irregular uterine cavity. Note abundant vascularity demonstrating residual placental tissue.

FETAL HEART

Color Doppler improves imaging of heart at all gestations. Crossing of great vessels can be demonstrated in approximately 51% at 10 weeks, improving to 90% at 11 weeks. IVC can be identified in 80% by 10 weeks.

FETAL DUCTUS VENOSUS

Ductus venosus can be identified with color Doppler and a waveform obtained by pulsed Doppler. It provides an independent contribution in the prediction of chromosomal abnormalities.[7] Abnormal ductus venosus flow increases the risk of cardiac defects in fetuses with nuchal translucency above 95th centile (Fig. 4.90). It may increase the risk in fetuses with normal nuchal translucency.[8] In monochorionic twins, abnormal flow in ductus venosus in at least one of the fetuses increases the risk of developing twin to twin transfusion (Figs. 4.91 to 4.93).[9]

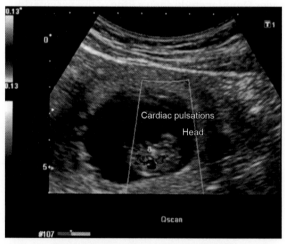

Fig. 4.90: Showing cardiac pulsations.

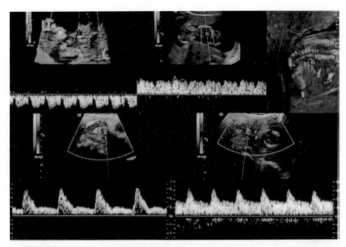

Fig. 4.91: Image shows normal flow at the ductus venosus with a positive wave. Blood flow at aortic arch and descending aorta. Fetal circulation can be imaged easily. Uterine artery color Doppler evaluation in the 1st trimester. Lower left picture shows uterine artery with notching and lower right shows normal uterine flow at diastole.

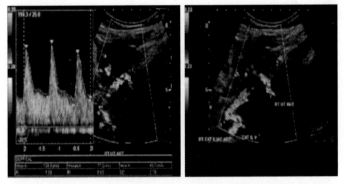

Fig. 4.92: The color Doppler ultrasound images show the uterine arteries on either side in a 14-week-old pregnancy.

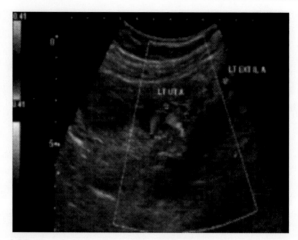

Fig. 4.93: Spectral waveform of the right uterine artery shows a normal early diastolic notch which is normally seen till the age of 25 weeks of gestation. PI and RI values early in the pregnancy can be quite high signifying increased resistance in the placental and chorionic, vascular beds. Thus PI values are typically higher than 2.5 in 11 to 14 week period, decreasing gradually as the gestation progresses. However, PI and RI values can vary depending on placental position (with low PI values in the uterine artery on the side of the placenta). Persistence of the diastolic notch and high PI and RI values can signify danger of the preeclampsia, placental abruption and PIH (pregnancy induced hypertension), and IUGR. Thus, uterine artery doppler can be used to predict or exclude danger to the fetus in the coming months. The left uterine artery in the color Doppler image above is smaller in size due to the placenta being more on the right side of the uterus.

PREDICTION OF PREECLAMPSIA

MoM values of uterine artery PI together with maternal characteristics and biochemical markers detection rate of up to 95% can be achieved in first trimester.[10] This will lead to potentially improved outcome of such patients by keeping them in surveillance.

REFERENCES

1. Barnett SB, Rott HD, Ter Haar GR, et al. The sensitivity of biological tissue to ultrasound. Ultrasound in Med and Biol. 1997;23:805-12.

2. ISUOG Bioeffects and Safety Committee; Safety statement, 2000 (reconfirmed 2002). Ultrasound Obstet Gynecol. 2002;19:105.

3. Cartier MS, Altieri LA, Emerson DS, et al. Diagnostic efficacy of endovaginal color flow Doppler in an ectopic pregnancy screening program. Radiology. 1990;177(p):117.

4. Dillon EH, Feyock AL, Taylor KJW. Pseudogestational sacs: Doppler US differentiation from normal or abnormal intrauterine pregnancies. Radiology. 1990;176:359-64.

5. Kurjak A, Zalud I, Predanic M, et la. Transvaginal and pulsed Doppler study of uterine blood flow in the first and early second trimesters of pregnancy: normal versus abnormal. J Ultrasound Med. 1994;13:43-7.

6. Ramanan RV, Gajaraj J, Ectopic pregnancy—the leash sign. A new sign on transvaginal Doppler ultrasound. Acta Radio. 2006;47:529-35.

7. Maiz N, Valencia C, Emmanuel EE, et al. Screening for adverse pregnancy outcome by ductus venosus Doppler at 11°–13+6 weeks of gestation.Obstet Gynecol. 2008;112:598-605.

8. Oh C, Harman C, Baschat AA. Abnormal first-trimester ductus venosus blood flow: a risk factor for adverse outcome in fetuses with normal nuchal translucency. Ultrasound Obstet Gynecol. 2007;30:192-6.

9. Maiz N, Staboulidou I, Leal AM, et al. Ductus venosus Doppler at 11–13 weeks of gestation in the prediction of outcome in twin pregnancies.Obstet Gynecol. 2009;113:860-5.

10. Akolekar R, Syngelaki A, Poon LC, et al. Competing risks model in early screening for preeclampsia by biophysical and biochemical markers. Fetal Diagn Ther. 2012.

4.25 EARLY FETAL ECHOCARDIOGRAPHY

Major congenital heart defects (CHDs) are the most common severe congenital malformations, with an incidence of approximately 5 per 1,000 live births. CHDs have a significant effect on life with up to 25–35% mortality rate during pregnancy and the post natal period and approximately 60% in first year of life. Major CHDs are responsible for nearly 50% of all neonatal and infant deaths due to congenital anomalies, and it is likely to be significantly higher if spontaneous abortions are considered.

Recently, the finding of an increased nuchal translucency[1,2] or an altered ductus venosus flow[3,4] at 10–14 weeks gestation have been associated with a high risk of CHD regardless of fetal karyotype. Their prevalence increases exponentially with the thickness of nuchal translucency. Cardiac defects diagnosed early in pregnancy tend to be more complex than those detected later on and use to cause more severe hemodynamic compromise in the developing fetus. With the help of high frequency TVS probes detailed study of cardiac structures at an early date is now possible. Application of color Doppler enhances the accuracy.

- The highest frequency must be used
- For color Doppler the energy levels have to be lower than 50 mW/cm² spatial peak temporal average.
- Four chamber view through transverse section of fetal chest is first assessed.
- Origin and double crossing of great arteries must be identified.
- The average duration of complete cardiac scan is 15 min.
- Best window of time is 13–16 weeks. Visualization up to 100% can be achieved at 13–14 weeks.

Diagnosis: First diagnosis was achieved by Gembruch[5] et al. in 1990, Bronchstein[6] et al. reported VSD at 14 weeks in same year (Fig. 4.94).

Indications

- Increased NT (>95th or 99th percentile)
- Abnormal ductus venosus flow regardless of NT

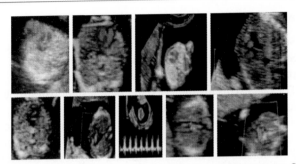

Fig. 4.94: Normal 4 chamber view at different gestational ages. Color Doppler evaluation of ventricular septum to diagnose VSD. Aortic outflow, pulmonary artery crossing over the aorta shown by color flow can be seen. Flow at the tricuspid valve can help us to diagnose chromosomal abnormalities at the 1st trimester. 3 vessel view showing normal outflow tract. Color flow also helps us to better visualize the outflow tracts.

- Fetuses affected by other structural malformations: hygroma, hydrops, omphalocele, situs inversus and arrhythmia.
- Multiple pregnancy with monochorionic placentation.
- Suspected cardiac anomalies at screening ultrasound
- Pregestational diabetes of mother
- High-risk family, with a previously affected child, first-degree relative with CHDs or a genetic disease in which CHDs are common
- Women at high risk of chromosomal abnormalities
- Pregnancies affected by chromosomal abnormality.

Advantages of Early Diagnosis

- The first benefit is early reassurance in high risk cases if everything is found normal
- Early diagnosis permits further testing like fetal karyotyping or in severe defects termination of pregnancy.
- In selected cases possibility of pharmacological therapy
- Correct timing and place of safe delivery may be planned.

Disadvantages

- Substantial amount of operator experience is required
- Small size of fetal heart and small space for mobility of TVS probe are limiting factors.
- The biggest disadvantage is later manifestation of structural and functional changes in some CHD.
- Some cardiac lesions are progressive and some obstructive lesions result in restricted growth of chambers or arteries.
- Few defects like muscular VSD are diagnosed which can otherwise resolve spontaneously in later pregnancy.

CONCLUSION

After a normal early echocardiography a conventional transabdominal echocardiography at 20–22 weeks is strongly recommended. Clinical follow-up in the neonate and postmortem examination, in those cases where termination of pregnancy is undertaken, are essential to assess the actual role of early echocardiography.

REFERENCES

1. Hyett J, Perdu M, Sharland G, et al. Using nuchal translucency to screen for major cardiac defects at 10–14 weeks of gestation:Population based cohort study. Br Med J. 1999;318: 81-5.
2. Devine PC, Simpson LL. Nuchal translucency and its relationship to congenital heart disease. Semin Perinatal. 2000;24: 343-51.
3. Matias A, Huggon I, Areias JC, et al. Cardiac defects in chromosomally normal fetuses with abnormal ductus venosus flow at 10–14 weeks. Ultrasound Obstet Gynecol. 1999;14:307-10.
4. Bilardo CM, Muller MA, Zikulnig L, et al. Ductu venosus studies in fetuses at high risk for chromosomal or heart abnormalities: Relationship with nuchal translucency measurement and fetal outcome. Ultrasound Obstet Gynecol. 2001;17:288-94.

5. Gembruch U, Knopfle G, Bald R, et al. Early diagnosis of fetal congenital heart disease by transvaginal echocardiography. Ultrasound Obstet Gynecol. 1993;3:310-17.
6. Bronshtein M, Zimmer EEZ, Gerlis LM, et al. Early ultrasound diagnosis of congenital heart defects in high risk and low risk pregnancies. Obstet Gynecol. 1993;82:225-29.

4.26 FIRST TRIMESTER CERVICOMETRY

Identification of women at high risk of preterm delivery by the end of first trimester, in place of second trimester, is of great interest in obstetrics, as it could give the opportunity for early intervention and plan effective strategy for prevention of greatest obstetric complication, i.e. preterm delivery.

Greco et al. proposed a new method for measuring cervical length in 1st trimester, making a distinction between the endocervix and the isthmus[1,2] which appears as a myometrial thickening between the endocervix and gestational sac. They suggested that what should be measured is first the linear distance between the two ends of the glandular area around the endocervical canal (endocervical length) and second the shortest distance between the glandular area and the gestational sac (isthmic length), distinguishing between the endocervix and the isthmus (Figs. 4.95A and B).

They studied 1,492 women and found that endocervical length is shorter in pregnancies resulting in spontaneous delivery before 34 weeks than in those delivering after 34 weeks. They could not find any difference if whole cervicoisthmic length was taken into consideration.

Following this study Souka et al also studied 800 women on same criteria and found prediction of preterm delivery before 34 weeks. (odds ratio 0.746; 95% confidence interval 0.649-0.869) and preterm delivery before 32 weeks (odds ratio, 0.734; 95% confidence interval, 0.637-0.912).[3,4]

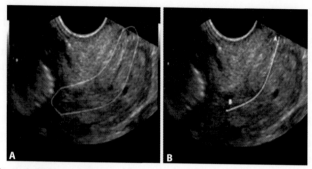

Figs. 4.95A and B: Transvaginal ultrasound pictures illustrating (A) The cervico-isthmic complex and (B) The measurement of the length of the endocervix.

CONCLUSION

With modern ultrasound machines and TVS, it is now possible to predict preterm labor by the end of 1st trimester in many, if not all the cases and take due steps to save those pregnancies.

REFERENCES

1. Greco E, Lange A, Ushakov F, et al. Prediction of spontaneous preterm elivery from endocervical length at 11 to 13 weeks. Prenat Diagn. 2011;31(1):84-9.
2. Greco E, Gupta R, Syngelaki A, et al. First-Trimester Screening for Spontaneous Preterm Delivery with Maternal Characteristics and Cervical Length. Fetal Diagn Ther. 2012.
3. Souka AP, Papastefanou I, Michalitsi V, et al. Cervical length changes from the first to second trimester of pregnancy, and prediction of preterm birth by first-trimester sonographic cervical measurement. J Ultrasound Med. 2011;30(7):997-1002.
4. Souka AP, Papastefanou I, Michalitsi V, et al. A predictive model of short cervix at 20–24 weeks using first-trimester cervical length measurement and maternal history. Prenat Diagn. 2011;31(2):202-6.

4.27 INVASIVE PROCEDURES IN FIRST TRIMESTER

Chorionic Villous Sampling

Ultrasound has an essential place in the performance of any invasive procedure and is important in avoiding damage to developing tissue. Chorionic villous sampling (CVS)[1] is a prenatal test in which a sample of chorionic villi is removed from the placenta for testing. Initial attempt was made in 1970s. It is usually done at 10–12 weeks.[2] CVS can reveal chromosomal disorders like Down syndrome, cystic fibrosis, Tay Sach's disease and more than 200 other disorders. As molecular genetics and gene defects leading to particular illnesses are now being identified, its demand has increased. It is also suitable for enzyme diagnosis.

Indications

- Positive prenatal screening tests by ultrasound, or biochemical or other method like NIPD.
- Chromosomal disorder in a previous pregnancy.
- Family history of genetic condition or chromosomal abnormality.
- Genetic condition in one of the parents.
- Advanced maternal age, risk is 1:400.[3] Other non-invasive tests should be done first.

  Procedure can be done transcervically or transabdominally.[4]

Procedure should not be done transcervically if:
- There is vaginal bleeding or spotting in previous two weeks
- Cervical infection
- Cervical stenosis
- Inaccessible placenta due to tilted uterus or growth in lower part of uterus.

Procedure should not be done transabdominally in:
- Acute retroversion of uterus and intestinal loops are coming in the way.
- Placenta is posterior with fetus obstructing the way.

Risks

- Miscarriage 1 in 100. Slightly higher for transcervical procedure 3–4.8%.[5]
- Rh sensitization: Rh immunoglobin should be administered if mother is Rh negative.
- Infections
- Amniotic fluid leakage resulting in hypoplastic lungs of fetus.
- Chances of defects in fingers and toes if done before 9 weeks.[6]

Chorionic villi and stem cells: They can be a rich source of multipotent mesenchymal stem cells (Fig. 4.96).[7]

Procedure

Transcervical: Polyethylene catheter app. Gauge 16 is used with malleable stainless steel obturator. Fetal membranes

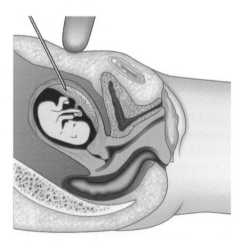

Fig. 4.96: Chorionic villus sampling: chorionic villi are aspirated transabdominally or transcervically using ultrasound guidance.

should be away from the tip. After removing obturator negative pressure is created by 20 mL syringe. The sample is transferred to transport media.

Transabdominal: Gauge 20 needle is used (single needle). In double needle technique 18 gauge needle is inserted, stillete removed, and a smaller 20 gauge needle with the syringe attached and moderate suction is applied. If tissue is insufficient previous needle can be used.

Limitations

- It cannot detect neural tube defects like spina bifida.
- 1–2% pregnancies have confined placental mosaicism, where some but not all placental cells tested in CVS are abnormal even though the pregnancy is unaffected.
- Cells from mother can be mixed with placental cells.[8]

Early Amniocentesis

The most common indication for genetic amniocentesis is prenatal diagnosis. Amniotic fluid can also be used for biochemical determinations, enzyme study and DNA hybridization.

Classically genetic amniocentesis is done in 2nd trimester. Early amniocentesis has all the advantages of early diagnosis but a significantly higher fetal loss rate (2–6%). Several studies have also reported an increased risk of congenital foot deformities,[9] mainly telepes equinovarus (1.6%). The yield of fetal cells is also less at this gestation.[10] In 1996, a new filtration technique for aspiration and culture of amniotic fluid in cases of early attempt was reported. The success in obtaining fetal cells was higher and mosaicism less.[11]

There is only one large Canadian study, early and mid trimester amniocentesis trial (CEMAT) published in 1998 showed 4 fold risk of technical difficulty (twice the risk of requiring multiple needle insertions), unsuccessful procedures

(1.6% vs. 0.4%),[10] fold risk of chromosomes culture failure (2.4 vs. 0.25%),[12] a higher rate of fluid leakage following procedure (3.5% vs. 1.7%), a greater risk of pregnancy losses (7.6% vs. 5.9%)[13] and a significantly higher risk of having a baby with telepes equinovarus (Fig. 4.97). The technical problem comes in the form of tenting due to amnion and chorion not being fused so early. Tenting occurs in 29.4% of DS v/s 8.3% in normal pregnancies.

Technique: A 20 gauge needle is guided into correct position, one hand holding transducer and app. 15 mL. amniotic fluid is aspirated.

Management of Ectopic Pregnancies

Local injection of methotrexate under ultrasound guidance is done laparoscopically or transvaginally. Use of color Doppler increases the success rate, as area of maximum color signal marks trophoblastic invasiveness and vitality.

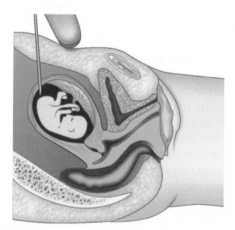

Fig. 4.97: Amniocentesis: Amniotic fluid cells are aspirated transabdominally using ultrasound guidance.

Multifetal Pregnancy Reduction (MFPR)

Multiembryonic conception and multifetal pregnancy are unwanted results of ART, with its attendant maternal, fetal and neonatal complications. It is very difficult decision to abort desperately wanted pregnancy. A pragmatic solution to this un-nerving problem and a promising way out of this medical-ethical-social pitfall is reducing the number of embryos.

The procedure is usually called multifetal pregnancy reduction (MFPR),[14] but as the procedure is generally performed in 1st trimester, it is a multiembryonic reduction.

Berkowitz, Evans and group published the first series of first trimester selective reduction of multifetal pregnancies in 1988. This procedure can be done by

- Transcervical suction
- Transvaginal aspiration
- Percutaneous transabdominal KCl inj. into thorax of the embryo. All under ultrasound guidance. The last procedure has been shown to be the best. 1–2 mL of 10% Kcl injected into the heart or thorax of embryo/fetus results in cardiac standstill in 1–2 minutes.
- Embryo to be eliminated should be easiest to reach.
- Should not be one near the cervix
- High order multiembryonic reduction should be done in two separate sittings.
- Reducing twins to singleton is not medically justified except in a woman with uterine malformation or significant medical disease like cardiac failure.
- World's largest centres suggest a 2% short term & 8% long term loss rate.

REFERENCES

1. Hahneman N. Possibility of culturing fetal cells at early stages of pregnancy. Clin Genet. 1972;3:286-93.
2. Alfirevic Z, van Dadelszen P. Alfirevic, Zarko, ed. "Instruments for Chorionic Villus Sampling for Prenatal diagnosis". Cochrane Database Syst Rev. 2003;(1): CD000114.
3. Incidence of Down syndrome in Pregnancy
4. Bettleheim D, Kolinek B, Schaller A, et al. Complication rates of invasive intrauterine procedures in a center for prenatal diagnosis and therapy. Ultrashall Med. 2002;119-22.
5. WHO/EURO Document EUR/ICP/MCH 123 Risk Evaluation of CVS. Copenhagen: World Health Organization Regional Office for Europe,1994.
6. Froster UG, Jackson L. Limb defects and chorionic villus sampling: results from an international registry1992-1994. Lancet. 1996;347:489-94.
7. Weiss, Rick. "Scientists See Potential In Amniotic Stem Cells". The Washington Post. Retrieved 2010-04-23.
8. Wapner, Ronald . "Invasive prenatal diagnostic techniques". Seminars in Perinatology. December 2005;29(6):401-4. doi: 10.1053/j.semperi.2006.01 .003.PMID 16533654
9. Nikkila A, Valentin L, Thelin A, Jorgensen C. Early amniocentesis and congenital foot deformity. Fetal Diagn Ther. 2002;17:129-32.
10. Golbus MS, Loughman WD, Epstein CJ, et al. Prenatal genetic diagnosis in 3000 amniocentesis. N Engl J Med. 1979;300:157.
11. Sundberg K, Lundsteen C, Phillip J. Comparison of cell cultures, chromosome quality and karyotypes obtained after chorionic villus sampling and early amniocentesis with filter technique. Prenat Diagn. 1997;19:12-16.
12. The Canadian Early and Mid-Trimester Amniocentesis Trial (CEMAT) Group 1998: Randomized trial to asses safety and fetal outcome of early and mid trimester amniocentesis. Lancet. 1998;351:242-47.
13. Rooney DE, Mac Lachlan N, Smith J, et al. Early amniocentesis: a cytogenetic evaluation. BMJ. 1989;299:25.
14. American College of Obstetricians and Gynecologists Ethics Statement: Committee on ethics. Multifetal pregnancy reduction and selective fetal termination. Int J Gynecol Obstet. 1992;38:140-2.

4.28 SCREENING FOR PREECLAMPSIA IN FIRST TRIMESTER

Effective screening for preeclampsia can be achieved by a combination of maternal characteristics and history, which constitutes a prior risk, combined with biophysical and biochemical markers. The uterine artery PI and MAP constitute the biophysical markers whereas maternal serum PAPP-A and PIGF are the biochemical markers. As demonstrated by the MoM values of uterine artery PI, MAP and serum PAPP-A and PIGF in pregnancies with PE, the distribution with gestational age is linear (Figs. 4.98 and 4.99).

In screening for PE requiring delivery before 34 weeks the detection rate, at a false positive rate of 10%, was about 50% by maternal characteristics and this was improved to 75% by the addition of biochemical markers and 90% by the addition of biophysical markers. The detection rate improved to more than 95% by an algorithm combining maternal factors, biophysical markers and biochemical markers.[1]

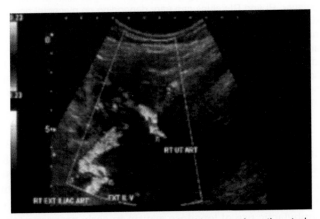

Fig. 4.98: The color Doppler ultrasound images show the uterine arteries on either side in a 14-week-old pregnancy.

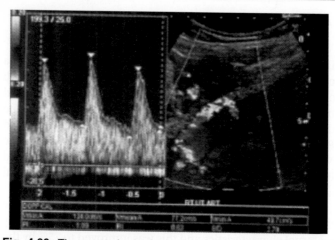

Fig. 4.99: The spectral waveform of the right uterine artery shows a normal early diastolic notch which is normally seen till the age of 25 weeks of gestation. PI and RI values early in the pregnancy can be quite high signifying increased resistance in the placental and chorionic vascular beds. Thus, PI values are typically higher than 2.5 in 11 to 14 week period, decreasing gradually as the gestation progresses. However, PI and RI values can vary depending on placental position (with low PI values in the uterine artery on the side of the placenta). Persistence of the diastolic notch and high PI and RI values can signify danger of the pre-eclampsia, placental abruption and PIH (pregnancy induced hypertension), and IUGR. Thus uterine artery doppler can be used to predict or exclude danger to the fetus in the coming months. The left uterine artery in the color Doppler image above is smaller in size due to the placenta being more on the right side of the uterus.

The use of an effective screening test for PE in the first trimester will allow for an accurate identification of a high risk group for subsequent development of PE. This will lead to a potentially improved outcome by directing such patients to specialist clinics for close surveillance and institution of prophylactic use of low dose aspirin in early pregnancy that can potentially halve the incidence of preeclampsia.[2, 3]

REFERENCES

1. Akolekar R, Syngelaki A, Poon LC, et al. Competing risks model in early screening for preeclampsia by biophysical and biochemical markers. Fetal Diagn Ther. 2012.
2. Bujold E, Roberge S, Lacasse Y, Bureau M, Audibert F et al. Prevention of preeclampsia and intrauterine growth restriction with aspirin started in early pregnancy: a meta- analysis. Obstet Gynecol. 2010;116:402-16.
3. Nicolaides KH. Turning the pyramid of prenatal care. Fetal Diagn Ther. 2011;29:183-96.

5

Second Trimester

5.1 INDICATIONS

- Follow-up observation of identified fetal anomaly or history of previous congenital anomaly
- Adjunct to amniocentesis
- Abnormal serum alpha-fetoprotein value
- Suspected polyhydramnios or oligohydramnios
- Advanced maternal age
- Exposure to drugs/radiation
- Maternal diabetes mellitus
- Bad obstetric history.

Scanning is done with a fully distended maternal bladder, though this is not essential after 20 weeks.

5.2 FETAL EVALUATION

- Number
- Fetal position especially in the late second trimester
- Viability
- Movements
- Gestational age
- Biometry.

5.3 FETAL EVALUATION (MALFORMATIONS)

The ideal way is to do a basic survey of fetal anatomy done systematically followed by a targeted fetal anatomy survey.

- Cranium
- Spine
- Neck
- Face
- Thorax and heart
- Abdomen
- Extremities.

5.4 CRANIUM (FIGS. 5.1 TO 5.39)

- Skull
- Brain
- Choroid plexus
  - Cysts
  - Hydrocephalus.
- Posterior cranial fossa
  - Cerebellar transverse diameter
  - Depth of cisterna magna
  - Superior and inferior cerebellar vermis
  - Posterior fossa cyst.
- Communication between fourth ventricle and cisterna magna.

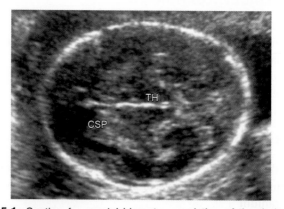

Fig. 5.1: Section for cranial biometry consisting of the thalamus, the third ventricle and the cavum septum pellucidum. The bi-parietal diameter is the side to side measurement from the outer table of the proximal skull to the inner table of the distal skull. The head perimeter is the total cranial circumference, which includes the maximum anteroposterior diameter. The occipito-frontal diameter is the front to back measurement from the outer table on both sides. (TH: Thalamus; CSP: Cavum septum pellucidum).

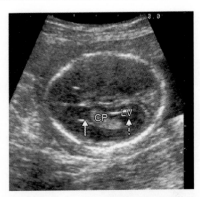

Fig. 5.2: Choroid plexus (CP) seen occupying the whole of the body of the lateral ventricle (LV). The anterior horn of the lateral ventricle (solid arrow) seen on the left side and posterior horn of the lateral ventricle (dashed arrow) seen on the right side are not filled by the choroid plexus. The choroid plexus quite often does not occupy the whole of the body of the lateral ventricle and the frontal and the posterior horn also are not filled by the choroids plexus. The width of the body of the lateral ventricle, the inter-hemispheric distance and the ratio of the width of the body of the lateral ventricle to the inter-hemispheric distance is calculated (Normal value <50%). This is not sensitive for early hydrocephalus. The width of the body, anterior horn and posterior horn of the lateral ventricle are taken (Normal value <8 mm, Borderline 8–10 mm and >10 mm abnormal).

5.5 NUCHAL SKIN (FIGS. 5.40 TO 5.42)

- Thickness
- Septations
- Cystic hygroma (Fig. 5.43 to 5.46)

5.6 FETAL ORBITS AND FACE (FIGS. 5.47 TO 5.66)

- Hypo and hypertelorism
- Lips
- Lens
- Nostrils
- Ear.

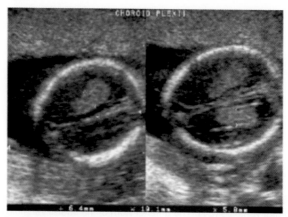

Fig. 5.3: When the choroid plexus does not occupy the whole of the body of the lateral ventricle see for the measurement of the medial separation of the choroid plexus from the wall of the lateral ventricle (Normal value <2 mm, Borderline 2–3 mm and >3 mm is abnormal).

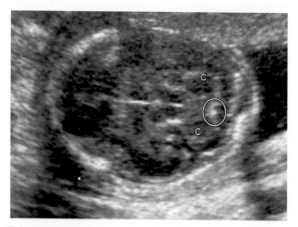

Fig. 5.4: The cerebellum is seen as a 'W' turned 90 degrees. The cerebellar hemispheres (C) and the cerebellar vermis (within the circle) should be appreciated for posterior cranial fossa abnormalities.

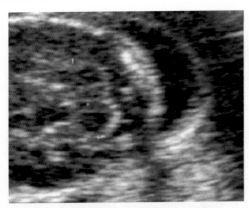

Fig. 5.5: The cerebellar transverse diameter (CTD) is measured from the edges of both cerebellar hemispheres. The CTD in mm from 14–22 weeks is equal to the gestational age of the fetus in weeks.

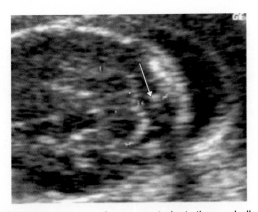

Fig. 5.6: The cisterna magna is seen posterior to the cerebellar vermis and anterior to the occipital bone (arrow). (Normal value <8 mm, Borderline 8–10 mm and >10 mm abnormal). Few strands seen traversing the cisterna magna are normal. Carefully check for any communication between the fourth ventricle and the cisterna magna with an abnormal cerebellar vermis. If there is any communication at gestational age less than 16 weeks reevaluate the fetus after 2 weeks.

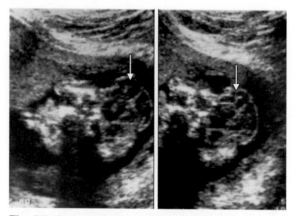

Fig. 5.7: Deformed cranium with almost no osseous area surrounding the floating brain (arrow).

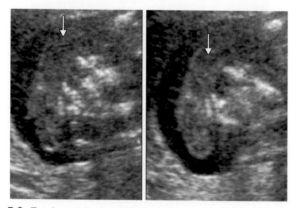

Fig. 5.8: Fetal acrania. Note the brain tissue (arrow) but no osseous covering over it.

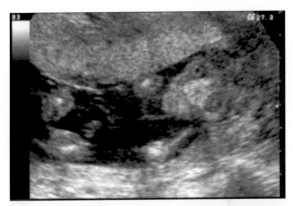

Fig. 5.9: Orbits seen with nothing seen superior to it
(neither brain nor bone).

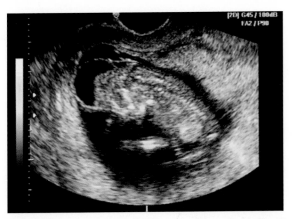

Fig. 5.10: Anencephaly: Superior to the orbits no brain tissue or
osseous portion is seen.

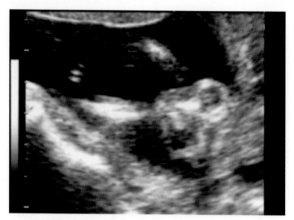

Fig. 5.11: Anencephaly with Toad sign.

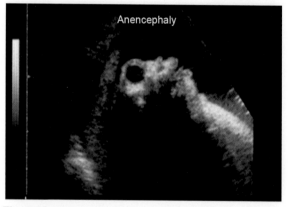

Fig. 5.12: Anencephaly with nothing superior to the orbits.

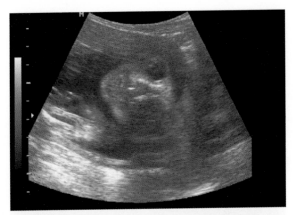

Fig. 5.13: Fetal face in an anencephalic fetus.

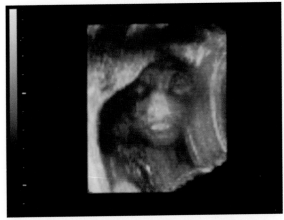

Fig. 5.14: Anencephaly as seen on 3D.

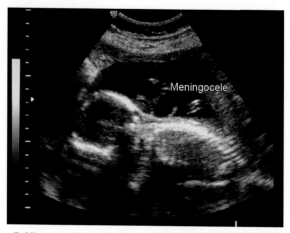

Fig. 5.15: Lateral occipital meningocele. Note the clear contents within the herniated sac.

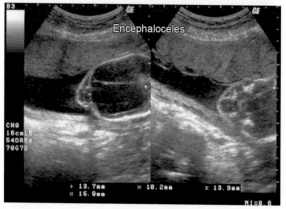

Fig. 5.16: Note the defect in the occipital bone with the herniation of brain tissue from the defect.

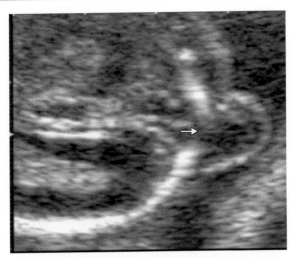

Fig. 5.17: Note the defect in the occipital bone (arrow) with the herniation of brain tissue from the defect.

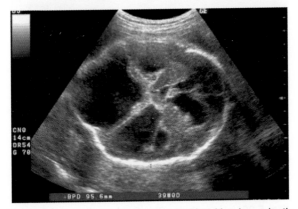

Fig. 5.18: Large occipital encephalocele with a hypoplastic cerebellar vermis.

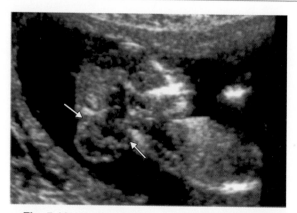

Fig. 5.19: Herniated contents (arrows) overhanging
the fetal neck.

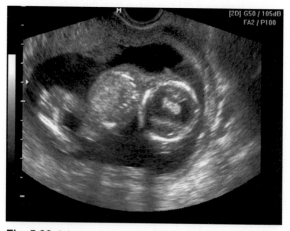

Fig. 5.20: Iniencephaly with a fixed retroflexion deformity
of the fetal head.

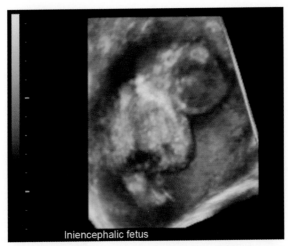

Iniencephalic fetus

Fig. 5.21: Iniencephaly as seen on 3D.

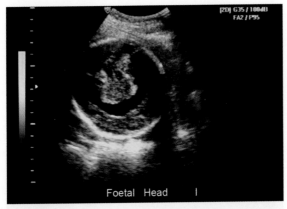

Foetal Head

Fig. 5.22: Alobar holoprosencephaly with a dorsal sac and a monoventricular cavity with a displaced cerebral cortex.

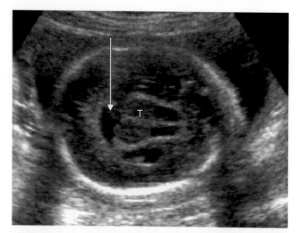

Fig. 5.23: Semilobar holoprosencephaly: Single primitive ventricle (holoventricle) (arrow) seen with thalami (T) fused in the midline.

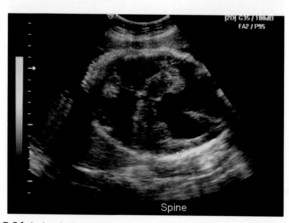

Fig. 5.24: Lobar holoprosencephaly: The septum pellucidum is absent but the inter-hemispheric fissure is well developed posteriorly.

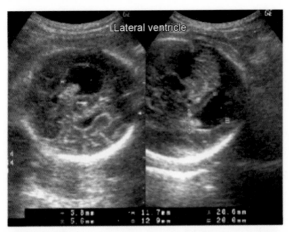

Fig. 5.25: Ventriculomegaly seen in the atrial and occipital regions (colpocephaly) because of poorly developed white matter surrounding these areas (Tear drop configuration) with an absent cavum septum pellucidum.

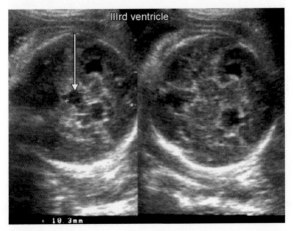

Fig. 5.26: An enlarged elevated third ventricle is seen between the hemispheres which appears as an interhemispheric cyst (arrow).

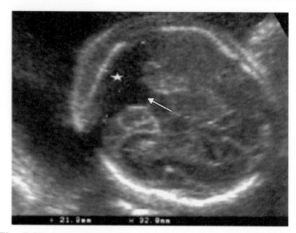

Fig. 5.27: Large cyst in the posterior cranial fossa (star) with a hypoplastic cerebellar vermis (arrow).

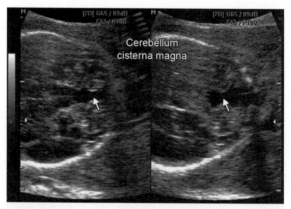

Fig. 5.28: Midline cyst in the posterior cranial fossa which is communicating (arrow) with the fourth ventricle.

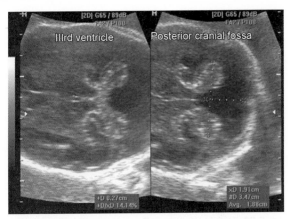

Fig. 5.29: Abnormally developed cerebellar vermis.

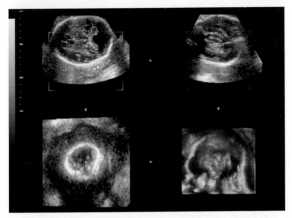

Fig. 5.30: Dandy Walker malformation as seen on
3D with all planes visualized.

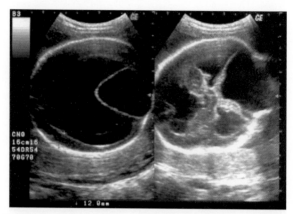

Fig. 5.31: Dandy-Walker malformation with hydrocephalus.

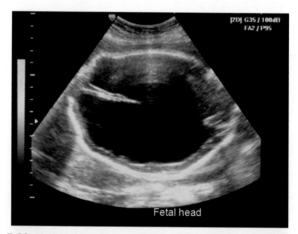

Fig. 5.32: Hydranencephaly with complete destruction of the cerebral cortex and basal ganglia with intact meninges and skull which is of normal appearance.

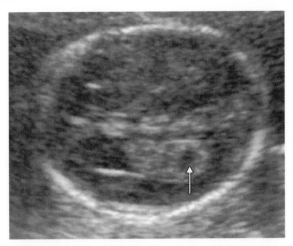

Fig. 5.33: Unilateral single (arrow) choroid plexus cyst.

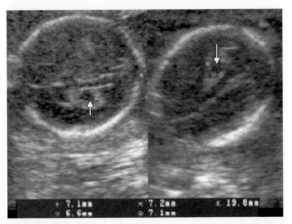

Fig. 5.34: Bilateral one on each side (arrow) choroid plexus cyst. A detailed scan to check for sonographic stigmata of chromosomal abnormalities especially Trisomy 18 is done and only if any additional anomaly is detected an amniocentesis is indicated for.

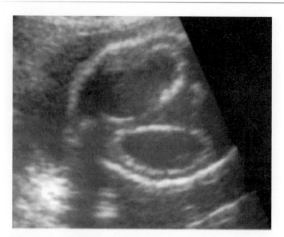

Fig. 5.35: Ventriculomegaly with hyperechoic walls and multiple foci of calcification seen in the brain substance.

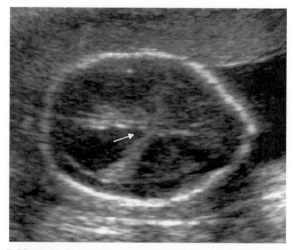

Fig. 5.36: Enlarged lateral ventricles with loss of the approximation between the choroid plexus and the medial border of the lateral ventricle (arrow).

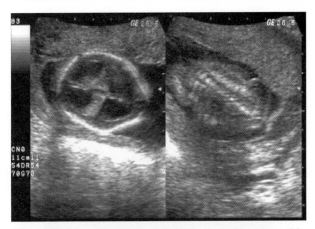

Fig. 5.37: Ventriculomegaly (left side) seen with a dysraphic disorganization of the lumbar and sacrococcygeal vertebrae.

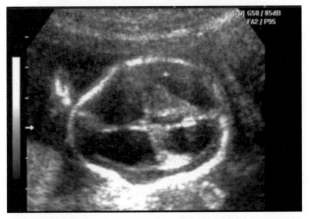

Fig. 5.38: Overlapping of the frontal bones seen in a case of communicating hydrocephalus.

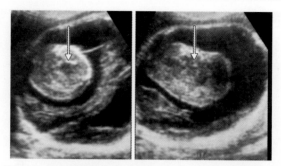

Fig. 5.39: Mass, possible a teratoma (arrows) with dilatation of the lateral ventricles.

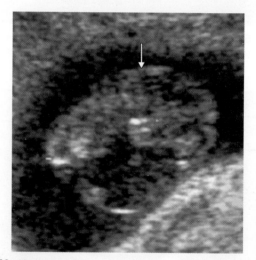

Fig. 5.40: Nuchal translucency in a 10 weeks fetus (arrow). Any thickening of the nuchal translucency prompts to a diagnosis of cystic hygroma, chromosomal abnormalities or cardiac abnormalities. Nuchal translucency in a 13 weeks fetus. Nuchal translucency thickness usually increases with gestational age with 1.5 mm and 2.5 mm being the 50th and 95th percentile respectively for gestational ages between 10 and 12 weeks. 2.0 mm and 3.0 mm are the 50th and 95th percentile respectively for gestational ages between 12 and 14 weeks.

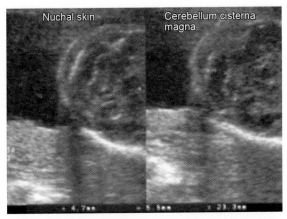

Fig. 5.41: Nuchal skin fold thickness assessment through the section for the cerebellum and cisterna magna.

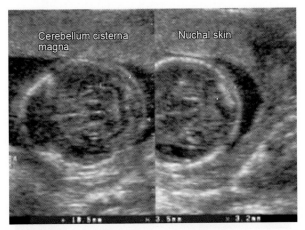

Fig. 5.42: Nuchal skin fold thickness assessment through the section just inferior to the section for cerebellum and cisterna magna. (14–18 weeks: Normal value <4 mm, Borderline 4–5 mm and >5 mm requires further karyotypic analysis) (18–22 weeks: Normal value <5 mm, Borderline 5–6 mm and >6 mm requires further karyotypic analysis).

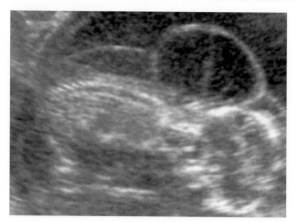

Fig. 5.43: Cystic hygroma seen in the longitudinal section across the entire fetal spine.

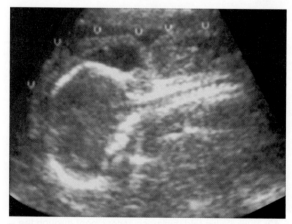

Fig. 5.44: Cystic hygroma seen in the longitudinal section posterior to the cranium, craniovertebral junction and cervical vertebra.

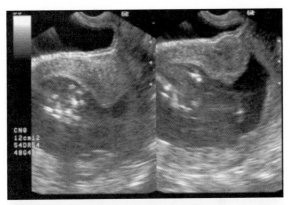

Fig. 5.45: Cystic hygroma seen as a diffuse lesion along the fetal thorax and abdomen.

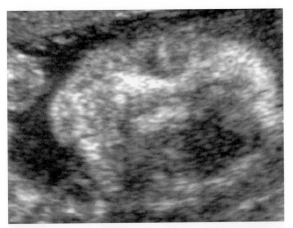

Fig. 5.46: Detailed facial anatomy which can be seen in a second trimester ultrasound. Note the eyelids, nose, lips, cheeks and chin which can be seen so clearly and can be shown to the expectant parents as well.

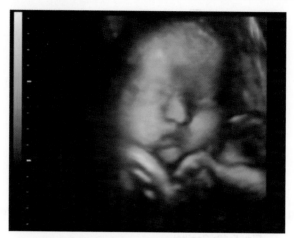

Fig. 5.47: Fetal face on 3D reconstruction.

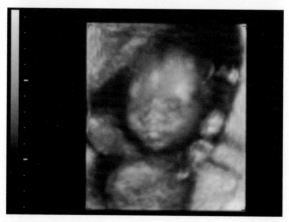

Fig. 5.48: Clear recognition of fetal facial features as seen on 3D.

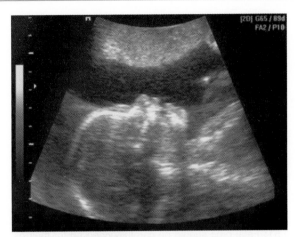

Fig. 5.49: Sagittal section through the mid-face showing the facial profile clearly.

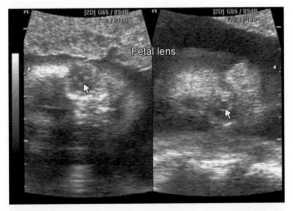

Fig. 5.50: Fetal lens seen in both the orbits on ultrasound is seen as a hyperechoic rim with a sonolucent center (arrow).

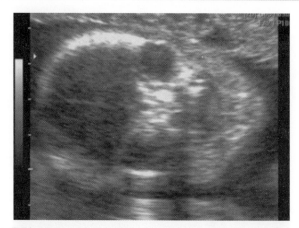

Fig. 5.51: Fetal orbit should be carefully checked for their osseous continuity apart from the measurements. View for the measurements of ocular diameter (measured from medial inner to medial lateral wall of the long orbit), interocular distance (measured from medial inner wall of one orbit to medial inner wall of the other orbit) and binocular distance (measured from lateral inner wall of one orbit to lateral inner wall of the other orbit).

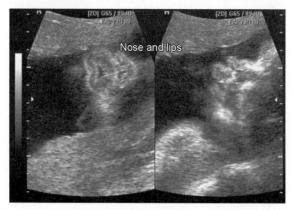

Fig. 5.52: Modified coronal view of the lower face showing the nostrils and the lips.

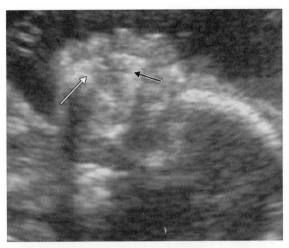

Fig. 5.53: Sagittal view showing the forehead, maxilla and mandible (arrow).

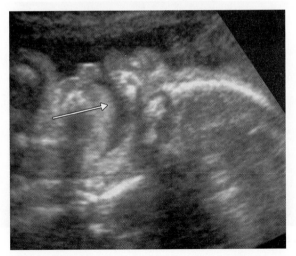

Fig. 5.54: Sagittal view of a normal fetal profile showing the osseous and soft tissue components. With the fetal mouth open the normal positioning of the tongue can also be seen.

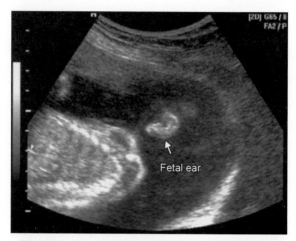

Fig. 5.55: Parasagittal view showing the external ear.

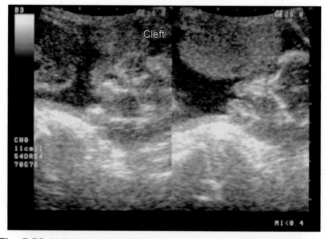

Fig. 5.56: Unilateral cleft lip extending into the maxilla as well.

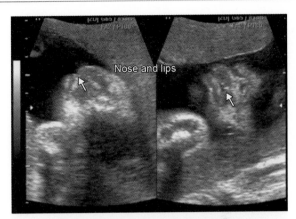

Fig. 5.57: Unilateral cleft lip (arrow).
Note the dropout of echoes in the upper lip.

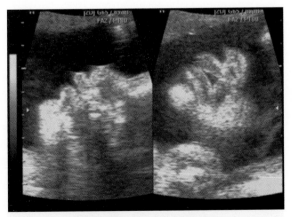

Fig. 5.58: Unilateral cleft lip.

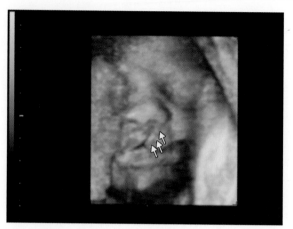

Fig. 5.59: 3D reconstruction of the cleft upper lip (arrow) as shown on 2D in Figure 5.58. This helps the parents to understand better.

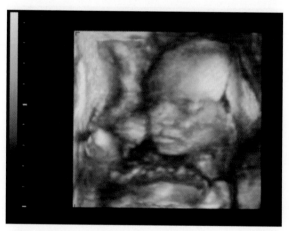

Fig. 5.60: 30 reconstruction of the bilateral cleft lip as seen from the side.

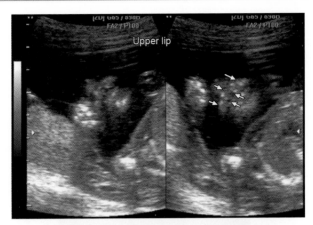

Fig. 5.61: Bilateral cleft lip and palate (arrows).

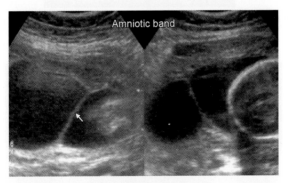

Fig. 5.62: Amniotic bands (arrow) can be associated
with a cleft lip or palate.

5.7 FETAL SPINE (FIGS 5.67 TO 5.79)

- Coronal
- Longitudinal
- Axial ossification
- Soft tissues.

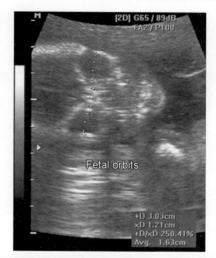

Fig. 5.63: Fetal orbits seen in the coronal view to assess for hypo/hypertelorism.

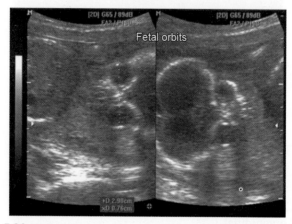

Fig. 5.64: Hypotelorism seen in a case of semilobar holopro-sencephaly. The ocular diameter in this case was 12 mm, the interocular distance was 8 mm and the binocular distance was 29 mm.

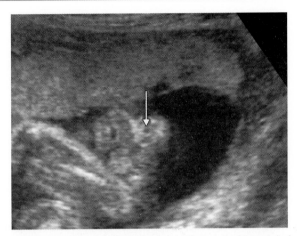

Fig. 5.65: Single nostril (arrow) seen in the case of hypotelorism with semilobar holoprosencephaly.

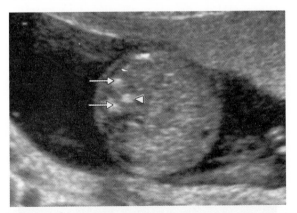

Fig. 5.66: Three ossification centers seen in the transverse planes. Two of these are posterior (arrows) and one is anterior (arrow head). Transverse planes to delineate any minimal widening of the interpedicular distance.

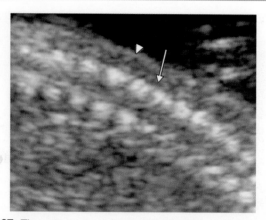

Fig. 5.67: The cutaneous, subcutaneous and muscular components seen posterior to the vertebral column all along the cervical, dorsal, lumbar and sacrococcygeal vertebrae (arrow and arrowhead). The longitudinal plane of the fetal spine delineating the soft tissues posterior to the vertebral column and any dysraphic disorganization of the spine.

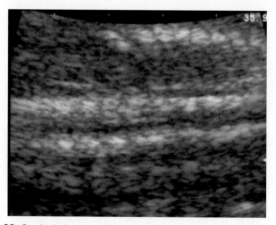

Fig. 5.68: Sagittal plane to delineate the spinal cord in the lower cervical, dorsal and lumbar spine and to delineate any osseous deformity.

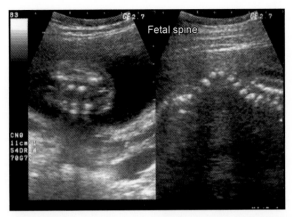

Fig. 5.69: Defect in the osseous component of the vertebral column and disruption of cutaneous and subcutaneous elements. Osseous disorganization of the fetal spine.

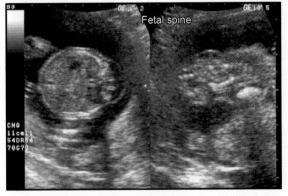

Fig. 5.70: Gross dysraphic disorganization of the entire spine.

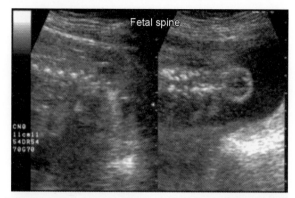

Fig. 5.71: Bulging membrane covering the vertebral lesion.

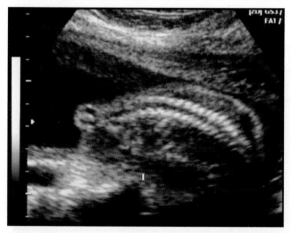

Fig. 5.72: Sacral meningocele with anechoic contents.

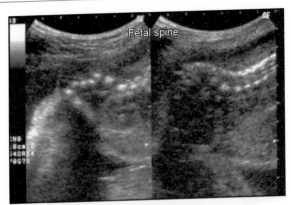

Fig. 5.73: Lumbosacral meningomyelocele.

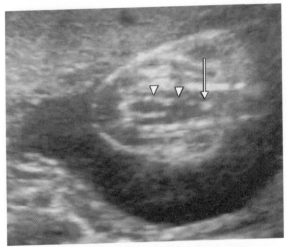

Fig. 5.74: Bony spicule (arrow) dividing the spinal cord (arrow heads).

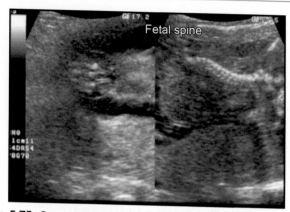

Fig. 5.75: Gross dysraphic disorganization of the entire fetal spine with a tethered spinal cord.

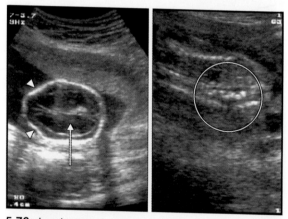

Fig. 5.76: Lumbosacral meningo-myelocele (within circle) with associated dilatation of the lateral ventricles (arrow) and frontal bossing (lemon sign) (arrow heads).

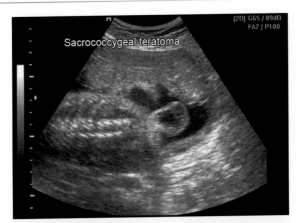

Fig. 5.77: Cystic sacrococcygeal teratoma.

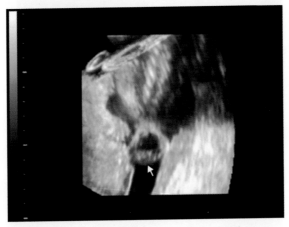

Fig. 5.78: 3D reconstruction of the postsacral mass.

5.8 FETAL THORAX (FIGS. 5.80 TO 5.95)

- Diaphragm
- Lung length

- Lung echoes
- Ribs
- Masses
- Cardiothoracic ratio.

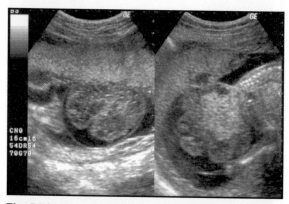

Fig. 5.79: Mass seen inferior to the sacrococcygeal area. Sacrococcygeal mass with a solid-cum-cystic echo pattern.

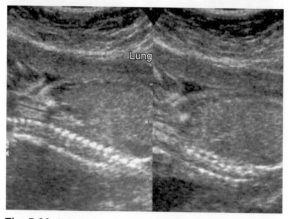

Fig. 5.80: Longitudinal section through the fetal thorax on both sides to assess the fetal lungs.

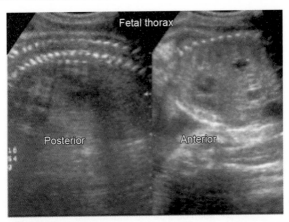

Fig. 5.81: Longitudinal section through the fetal thorax to assess the spine posteriorly (for osseous deformities, meningoceles or meningomyeloceles, anterior or posterior) and anterior thoracic wall anteriorly (for any thinning or ectopia cordis).

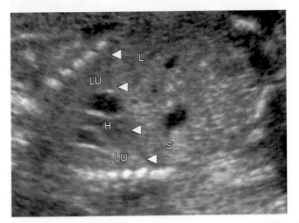

Fig. 5.82: Diffusely homogeneous fetal lung (LU) seen as diffuse low level echoes in comparison with the fetal liver (L). Diaphragm seen as arrow heads.

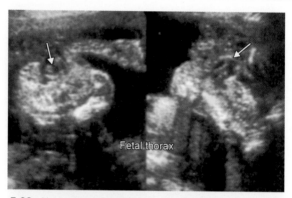

Fig. 5.83: Absent anterior thoracic wall with the fetal heart (arrow) seen outside the fetal thorax.

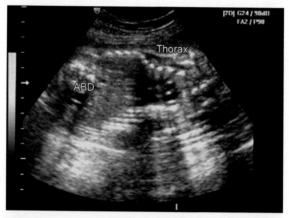

Fig. 5.84: Narrow fetal thorax in comparison with the fetal abdomen. (ABD: Abdomen)

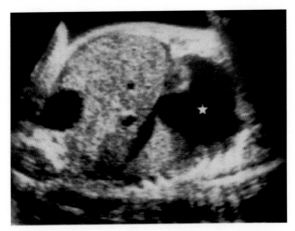

Fig. 5.85: Large pleural effusion (star) taking on the shape of the chest wall, diaphragm and mediastinal contour.

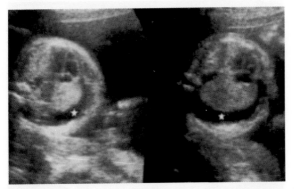

Fig. 5.86: Unilateral pleural effusion (star) taking the shape of the chest wall and mediastinum.

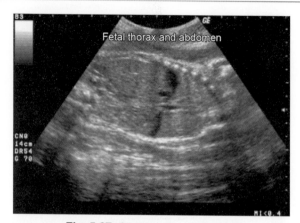

Fig. 5.87: Bilateral pleural effusion.

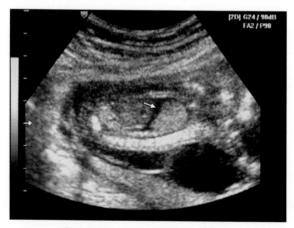

Fig. 5.88: Pleural effusion (arrow).

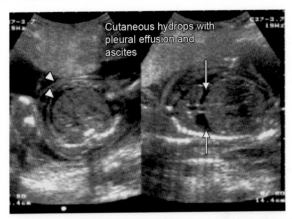

Fig. 5.89: Bilateral pleural effusion (arrow) as a part of generalized hydrops. Note the cutaneous hydrops over the abdominal wall and ascites (arrowheads).

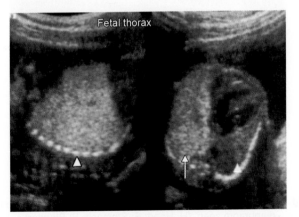

Fig. 5.90: Cystic adenomatoid malformation of the right lung (arrow). Because of distal acoustic enhancement from very small cysts the lesion appears as a solid mass. Note the difference in echo pattern from the left lung (arrow head).

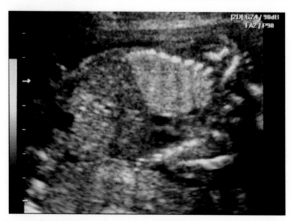

Fig. 5.91: Cystic adenomatoid malformation of the fetal lung.

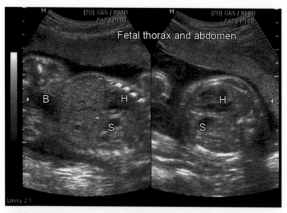

Fig. 5.92: Fetal stomach (S) seen in the retrocardiac area with the diaphragm seen. (H: Heart; S: Stomach; B: Bladder).

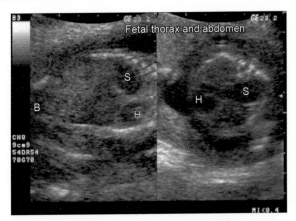

Fig. 5.93: Fetal stomach seen posterior to the fetal heart as seen in a longitudinal and transverse section. (H: Heart; S: Stomach; B: Bladder).

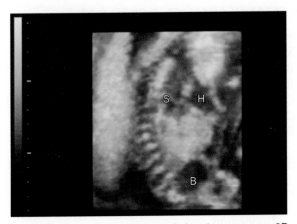

Fig. 5.94: Congenital diaphragmatic hernia as seen on 3D. (H: Heart; S: Stomach; B: Bladder).

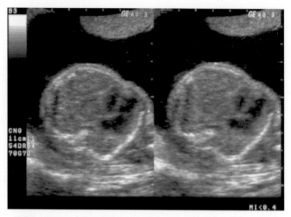

Fig. 5.95: Right sided diaphragmatic hernia. The mass is almost isoechoic with the lung.

5.9 FETAL HEART (FIGS. 5.96 TO 5.116)

- Situs
- Size
- Rate
- Rhythm
- Configuration
- Connections
- Fetal circulation.

5.10 FETAL ABDOMEN (FIGS. 5.117 TO 5.154)

- Gastrointestinal
  - Stomach
  - Duodenum
  - Small bowel
  - Large bowel
  - Omentum
  - Mesentery.

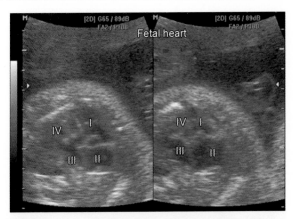

Fig. 5.96: Cardiac four-chamber view. Please note that with the spine lateral or posterior one can get a good four chamber view of the heart. (I: Right ventricle; II: Right atrium; III: Left atrium; IV: Left ventricle)

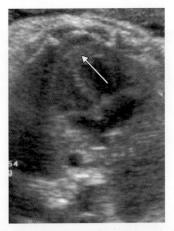

Fig. 5.97: Moderator band (arrow) seen in the right ventricle at the apex.

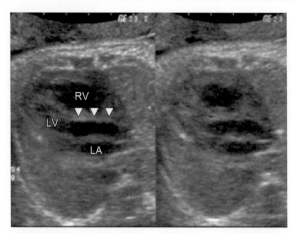

Fig. 5.98: Aortoseptal continuity (arrow heads) seen in the long axis view. The left ventricle (LV), right ventricle (RV) and left atrium (LA) are also labeled.

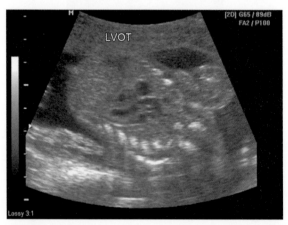

Fig. 5.99: Another view of the left ventricular outflow tract showing aortoseptal continuity. (LVOT: Left ventricular outflow tract).

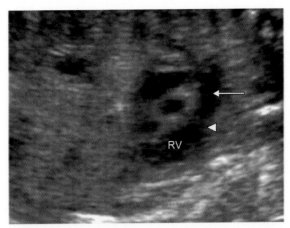

Fig. 5.100: Right ventricle (RV), pulmonary valve (arrowhead) and pulmonary artery (arrow) seen as the right ventricular outflow tract.

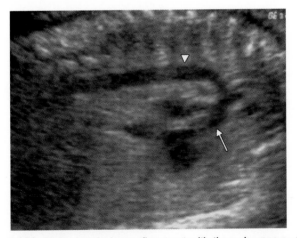

Fig. 5.101: Right ventricular outflow tract with the pulmonary artery (arrow) from the right ventricle going into the ductus arteriosus and descending aorta (arrowhead).

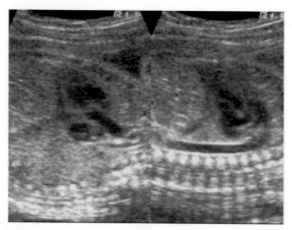

Fig. 5.102: Left ventricular outflow tract with aortoseptal continuity (left side) and right ventricular outflow tract with the pulmonary artery (right side) shown.

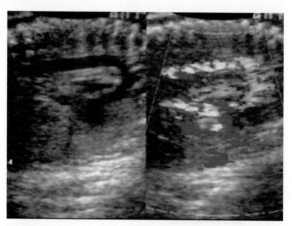

Fig. 5.103: Aortic arch seen from the fetal heart and its branches in the neck.

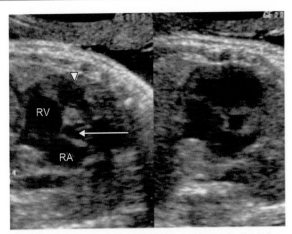

Fig. 5.104: Right atrium (RA), right ventricle (RV) and pulmonary artery (arrowhead) seen in the short axis view encircling the aorta (arrow).

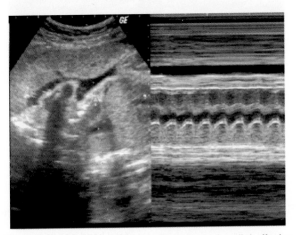

Fig. 5.105: M-mode tracings to check for pericardial effusion, chamber size and wall thickness.

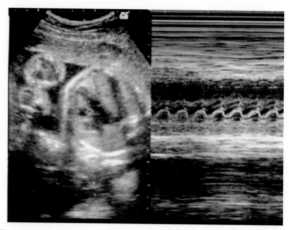

Fig. 5.106: M-mode tracings with the cursor through the right ventricle, left ventricle and left atrium.

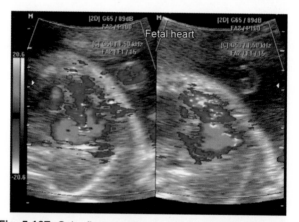

Fig. 5.107: Color flow mapping for assessing flow through the atrioventricular valves.

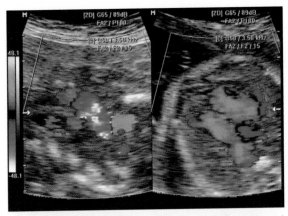

Fig. 5.108: Color flow mapping for assessing flow through and distal to the semilunar valves.

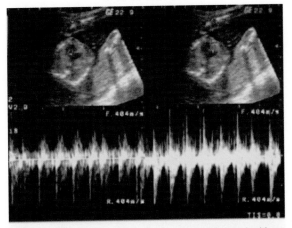

Fig. 5.109: Doppler gate for sampling for arterial flow velocities across the atrioventricular valves for peak flow velocities and volume flow across these valves for delineation of stenosis or regurgitation.

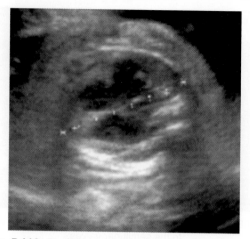

Fig. 5.110: Cardiomegaly with the cardiothoracic ratio in this case as 80%.

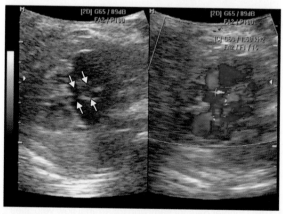

Fig. 5.111: Four chamber view with a large ventricular septal defect (arrows) and an atrial septal defect.

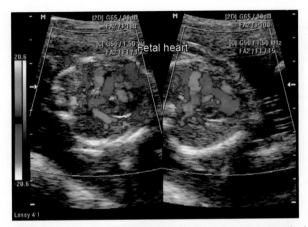

Fig. 5.112: Four chamber view with a perimembranous ventricular septal defect.

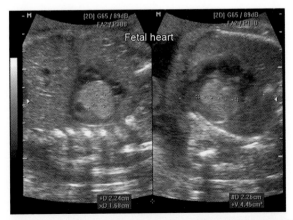

Fig. 5.113: Cardiac rhabdomyoma with a diffuse thickening of the myocardium.

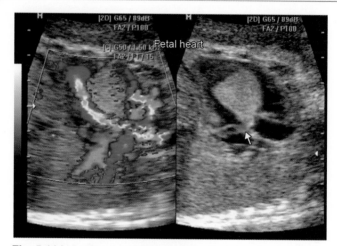

Fig. 5.114: Outflow tracts seen on color flow mapping around the rhabdomyoma.

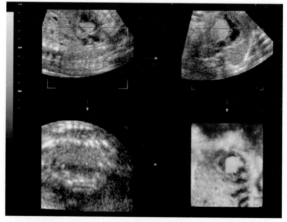

Fig. 5.115: Cardiac tumor as seen on 3D.

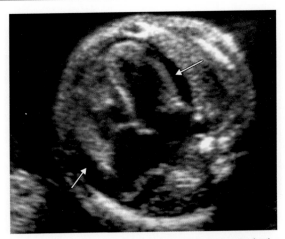

Fig. 5.116: Pericardial effusion (arrows) seen enveloping the fetal heart.

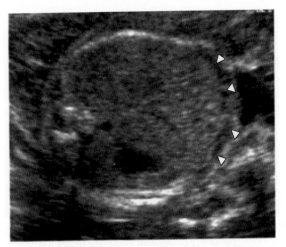

Fig. 5.117: Pseudoascites (arrow heads) is the hypoechoic area seen only along the anterior and lateral aspects on the periphery commonly seen in a transverse section.

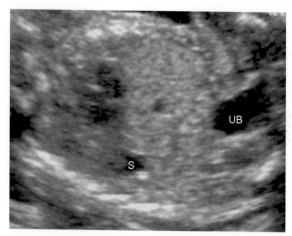

Fig. 5.118: Fluid filled structures, stomach (S) and urinary bladder (UB) seen in the fetal abdomen.

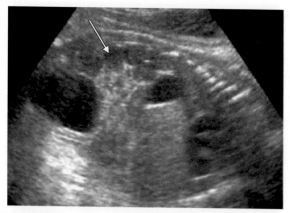

Fig. 5.119: Normal colonic echoes (hypoechoic) seen at the periphery of the fetal abdomen (arrow).

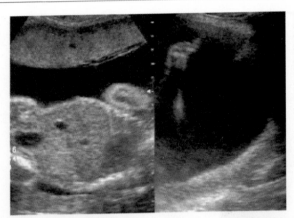

Fig. 5.120: Esophageal atresia as diagnosed by demonstration of polyhydramnios (right side) with an inability to visualize the stomach bubble (left side).

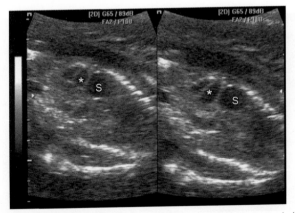

Fig. 5.121: Double bubble sign seen as a distended stomach (S) and an enlarged duodenal bulb (star).

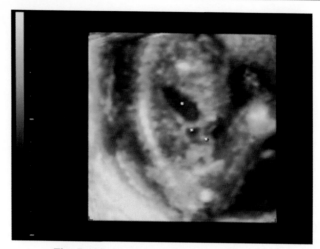

Fig. 5.122: Duodenal atresia as seen on 3D.

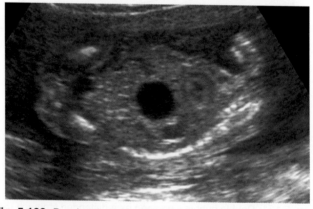

Fig. 5.123: Duodenal atresia with fetal stomach and duodenal bulb.

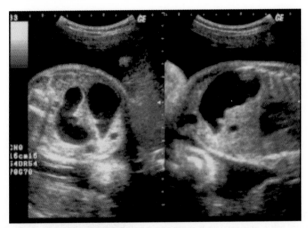

Fig. 5.124: Dilated stomach and duodenum.

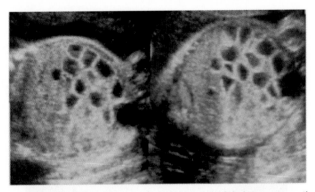

Fig. 5.125: Small bowel obstruction seen as multiple inter-connecting, overdistended bowel loops more than 7 mm in diameter. Take care that you do not confuse the same picture with a multicystic dysplastic kidney or a dilated tortuous ureter.

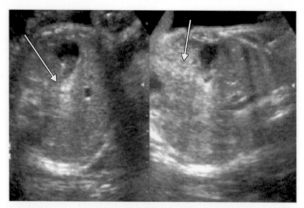

Fig. 5.126: Echogenic bowel (arrow) which can be normally seen in a normal fetus at term with hyperechoic colonic meconium or hyperechoic bowel contents in the fetus who has swallowed intraamniotic blood.

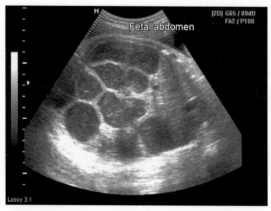

Fig. 5.127: Dilated large bowel segments seen near the periphery in a case of anorectal malformation.

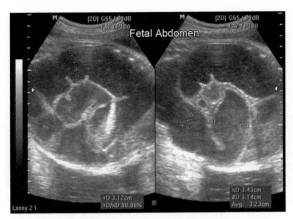

Fig. 5.128: Dilated large bowel loops (30–34 mm).

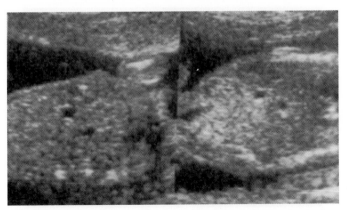

Fig. 5.129: Scattered echogenic foci with distal acoustic shadowing in a case of meconium peritonitis.

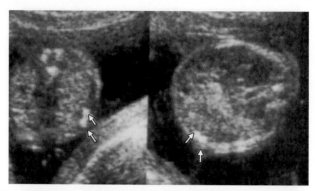

Fig. 5.130: Dense hyperechoic foci (arrows) seen in the periphery in a case of meconium peritonitis.

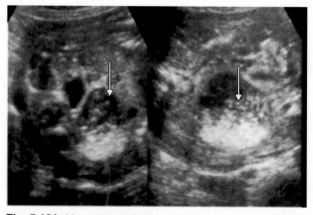

Fig. 5.131: Meconium peritonitis with a meconium pseudocyst (arrow) with debris seen within it.

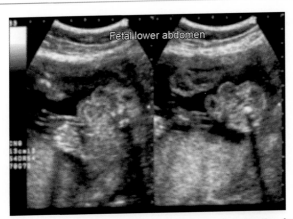

Fig. 5.132: Gastroschisis with bowel segments seen floating freely in the amniotic fluid.

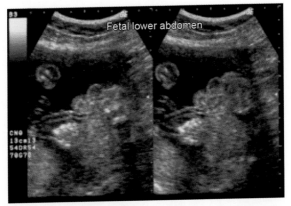

Fig. 5.133: Gastroschisis with bowel loops floating and on 2D ultrasound the umbilical cord is seen on the side of the lesion.

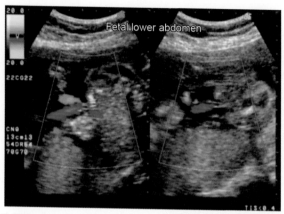

Fig. 5.134: Anterior abdominal wall defect (gastroschisis) with the umbilical cord insertion on the side of the lesion as seen on color flow mapping.

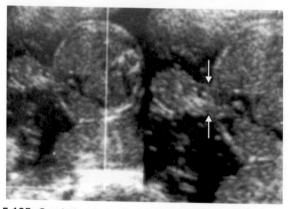

Fig. 5.135: Omphalocele (arrow) seen in a case of trisomy 18.

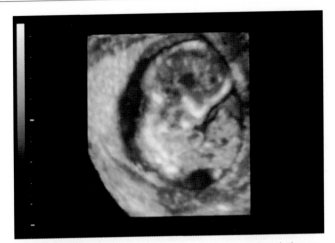

Fig. 5.136: Omphalocele with abdominal viscera herniating as seen on 3D.

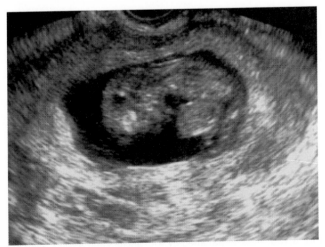

Fig. 5.137: Omphalocele in an early second trimester fetus.

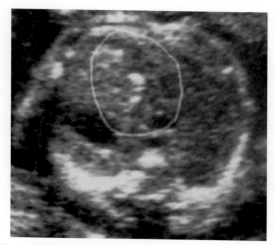

Fig. 5.138: Multiple foci of hepatic calcification in a case of intrauterine infection.

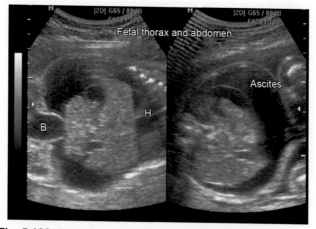

Fig. 5.139: Fetal hepatomegaly with ascites and ascites seen in a case of toxoplasmosis infection. (H: Heart; B: Bladder).

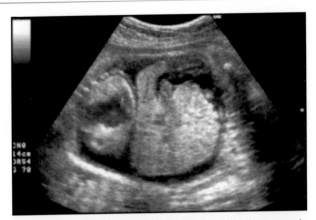

Fig. 5.140: Fetal hepatomegaly with gross fetal ascites seen in a case of severe fetal hydrops.

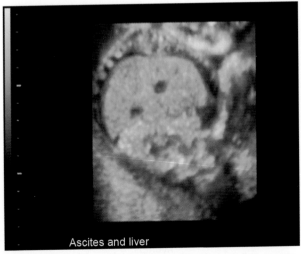

Fig. 5.141: Fetal hepatomegaly and ascites as seen on 3D.

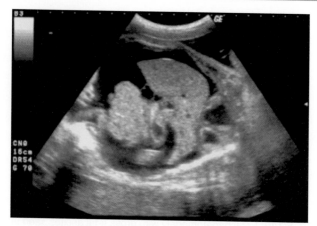

Fig. 5.142: Fetal hepatomegaly.

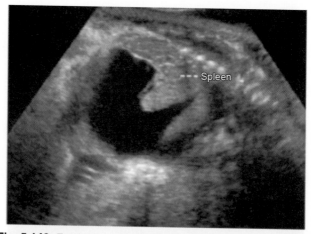

Fig. 5.143: Fetal splenomegaly (labeled) in a case of severe fetal hydrops.

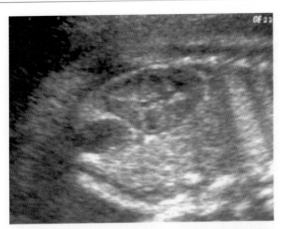

Fig. 5.144: Longitudinal scan of a normal kidney with its characteristic reniform shape.

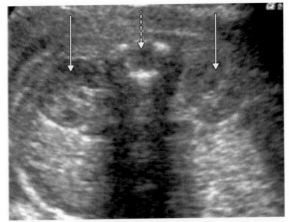

Fig. 5.145: Transverse section through the fetal abdomen showing both kidneys (arrow) on either side of the spine (dashed arrow).

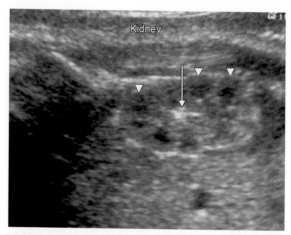

Fig. 5.146: Longitudinal scan of a normal kidney in the third trimester in a fetus of 33 weeks and 4 days. Note the central echogenic area (arrow) with hypoechoic pyramids (arrowheads).

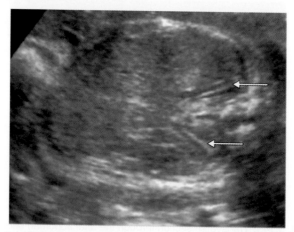

Fig. 5.147: Fetal adrenal glands as seen normally (arrow). Be careful not to mistake the adrenal for a kidney especially in cases of renal agenesis. To differentiate remember that the adrenal gland does not have central sinus echoes and a reniform shape.

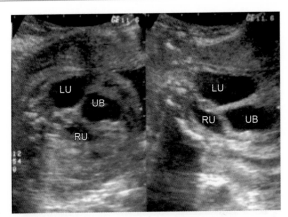

Fig. 5.148: Obstruction of the urinary tract at the bladder outlet with an overdistended urinary bladder, dilated ureters on both sides and a bilateral hydronephrosis. (UB: Urinary bladder; TU: Right ureter; LU: Left ureter).

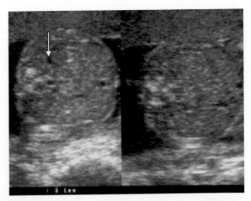

Fig. 5.149: Anteroposterior diameter of the renal pelvis (arrow). The values for the anteroposterior diameter of the renal pelvis (measured on a transverse view through the kidney) are from 15 to 20 weeks of gestation <4 mm is normal, 4 to 7 mm is borderline and >8 mm is abnormal or hydronephrotic. From 20 weeks onward <6 mm is normal, 6 to 9 is borderline and >10 mm is abnormal or hydronephrotic. Be careful that borderline cases are to be reviewed by serial scans before labeling them as hydronephrotic.

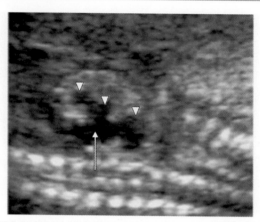

Fig. 5.150: Pelviureteric junction obstruction with a dilated renal pelvis (arrow) with dilated calyces (arrowheads). No ureteric dilatation is seen.

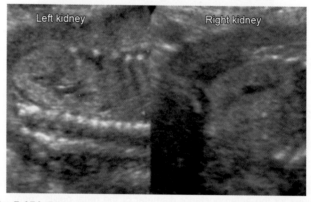

Fig. 5.151: Bilateral echogenic kidneys which are dysplastic and small with very less pelviectasis. This is not a reduction in hydronephrosis as the improvement with dysplastic kidney is because the renal function is poor or absent and is not going to improve even after the obstruction is corrected.

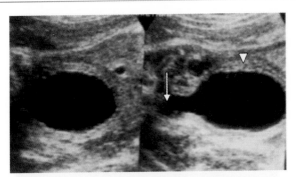

Fig. 5.152: Bladder outlet obstruction with dilatation of the proximal urethra (arrow) and a thickened urinary bladder wall (arrowhead).

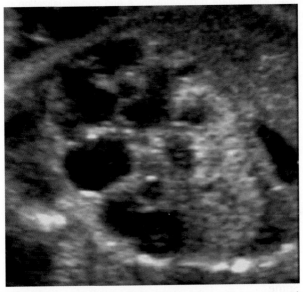

Fig. 5.153: Multicystic dysplastic kidney with multiple cysts and no normal renal parenchyma seen.

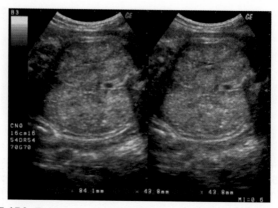

Fig. 5.154: Enlarged echogenic kidneys (infantile polycystic kidney disease) with severe oligohydramnios and non-visualization of the urinary bladder.

- Hepatobiliary
  - Liver
  - Gallbladder.
- Genitourinary
  - Kidneys
  - Ureters
  - Urinary bladder.
- Pancreas
- Spleen.

5.11 FETAL SKELETON (FIG. 5.155 TO 5.168)

- Cranium
- Mandible
- Clavicle
- Spine
- Extremities.

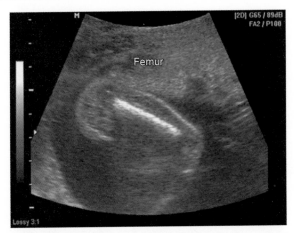

Fig. 5.155: Femoral length to be measured routinely in all obstetric ultrasound after 14 weeks. If a skeletal deformity is being suspected the tibial and fibular lengths also to be taken.

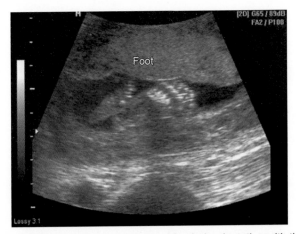

Fig. 5.156: Fetal feet to be checked for their orientation with the tibia to make a diagnosis of club foot.

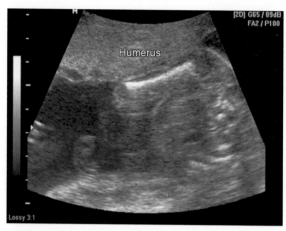

Fig. 5.157: Humeral length to be measured in all anomaly targeted obstetric ultrasound especially for chromosomal abnormalities after 14 weeks. If a skeletal deformity is being suspected the radial and ulnar lengths also to be taken.

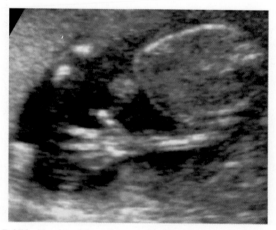

Fig. 5.158: Fetal hands to be checked for position, orientation and to look for polysyndactyly.

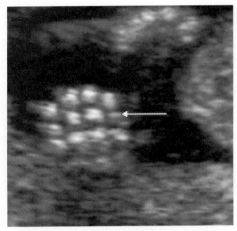

Fig. 5.159: The fifth digit should be carefully assessed for any incurving or any hypoplasia of the middle phalanx of the fifth digit (arrow).

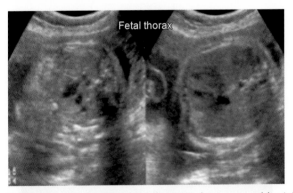

Fig. 5.160: Narrowing of the fetal thorax to be assessed by taking the thoracic perimeter and checking the abdominal perimeter/thoracic perimeter ratio. One should also assess by taking the maximum anteroposterior measurement of the thorax and the abdomen on a longitudinal section. Configuration of ribs to be seen on both sides to check for any thoracic narrowing with resultant pulmonary hypoplasia and a bad prognosis.

```
            MEAN( mm, mm² ) GA
BPD(CAM)    47.6      19w5d  ±1w0d
OFD(HAN)    58.3      19w4d  ±5.30mm
HC (HAD)   164.1      19w1d  ±1w3d
AC (HAD)   137.5      19w1d  ±2w0d
FL (HAD)    20.3      16w0d  ±1w3d
HUM(JEA)    20.3      16w0d  ±2w5d
RAD(MEZ)    13.9      15w3d  ±3.50mm
ULN(JEA)    15.2      15w1d  ±3w0d
TIB(JEA)    13.5      14w4d  ±2w6d
FIB(MEZ)    12.8      14w3d  ±3.00mm
THO(HAN)    32.0      16w0d  ±4.70mm
```

Fig. 5.161: Report on parameters of a case of thanatophoric dysplasia. Cranial parameters and abdominal perimeter correspond to 19–20 weeks size, thoracic dimensions to 16 weeks size and bone lengths to 14–15 weeks size.

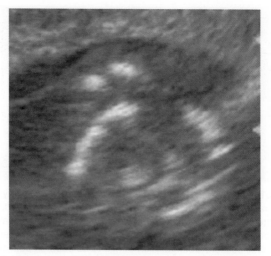

Fig. 5.162: Bowed long bones almost giving a telephone receiver appearance.

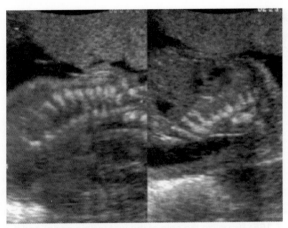

Fig. 5.163: Narrow thorax, in the longitudinal section compare the side to side measurement of the fetal thorax and abdomen.

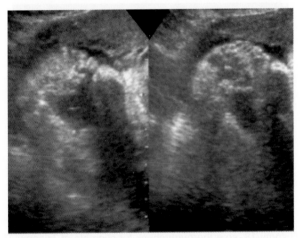

Fig. 5.164: Fetal foot turned medially in a case of club foot.

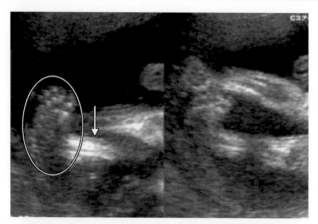

Fig. 5.165: Visualize the sole of the foot (within circle) and if in this view you can see the tibia (arrow) it is a club foot deformity.

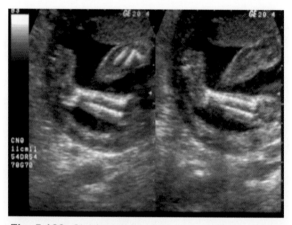

Fig. 5.166: Clubfoot deformity can be associated with Trisomy 18, so a thorough check for stigmata of Trisomy 18 should be done.

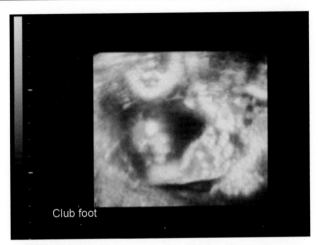

Club foot

Fig. 5.167: Clubfoot as seen on 3D reconstruction.

5.12 FETAL BIOMETRY

- Biparietal diameter
- Occipito frontal distance
- Head perimeter
- Abdominal perimeter
- Femoral length
- Humeral length.

5.13 EXTRA-FETAL EVALUATION

- Placenta (Location, morphology, focal lesions, retroplacental area) (Figs. 5.169 to 5.173)
- Liquor amnii (Normal, oligohydramnios, polyhydra-mnios, amniotic bands) (Figs. 5.174 to 5.177)
- Umbilical cord (Number of Vessels, Origin and insertion, Masses) (Figs. 5.178 to 5.182)

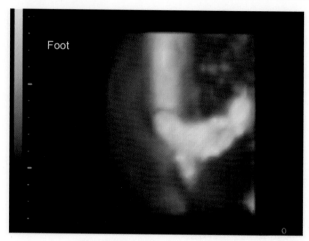

Fig. 5.168: 3D view of clubfoot.

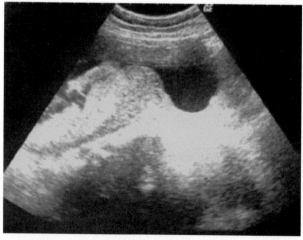

Fig. 5.169: An upper segment placenta as the placenta in this case is far away from the internal os.

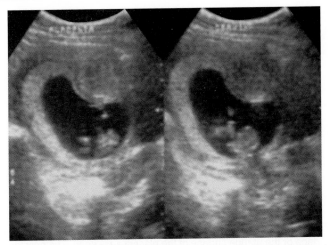

Fig. 5.170: The placenta is posterior. Its inferior limit extends down to the internal os but does not span across it.

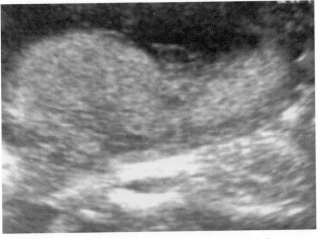

Fig. 5.171: Grade I placenta at 20 weeks and 2 days.

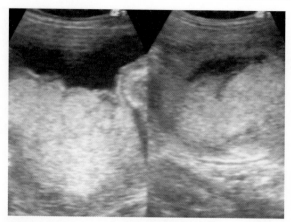

Fig. 5.172: Multiple anechoic or hypoechoic areas near the fetal surface or the uterine surface of the placenta are seen. The only focal lesion of significance is chorioangioma which is hypoechoic and very vascular.

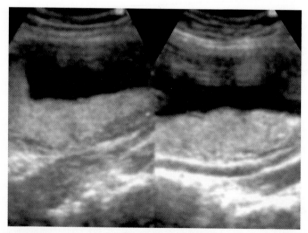

Fig. 5.173: The retroplacental area usually appears hypoechoic because of vessels, so do not mistake it as retroplacental collection.

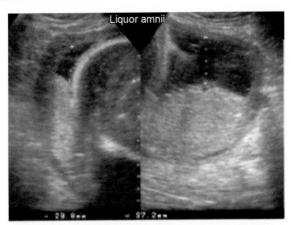

Fig. 5.174: Amniotic fluid index assessment. The uterus is divided into four quadrants by the midline and transverse axis and the amniotic fluid as the deepest vertical pocket free of fetal parts and umbilical cord is measured in each quadrant and all four quadrants add up to give the amniotic fluid index . Gradation of the amniotic fluid into oligopolyhydramnios is then done.

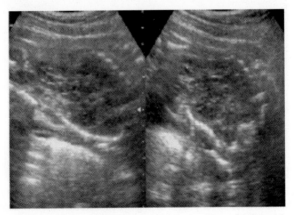

Fig. 5.175: Severe oligohydramnios in a case of bilateral renal agenesis. Note the complete absence of liquor amnii with the uterine wall closely apposed to the fetus.

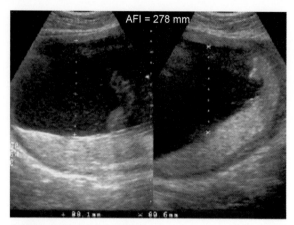

Fig. 5.176: Moderate polyhydramnios in a case of congenital diaphragmatic hernia. Diagnosis is striking in these cases as the fetus is seen freely mobile in liquor amnii. Both pockets shown in the picture are more than 80 mm each.

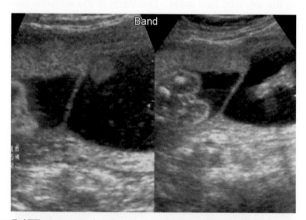

Fig. 5.177: Amniotic fold/band seen traversing the uterine cavity. Be careful to check for any limb or digit reduction/constriction defects, external anomalies of the face (cleft lip and palate, nasal abnormalities), cranium (anencephaly or encephalocele), anterior abdominal wall defects and abnormal curvature of the spine.

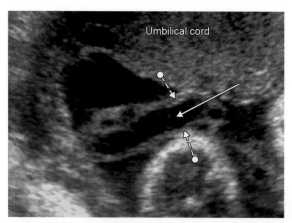

Fig. 5.178: Three vessel cord as seen on 2D ultrasound. The single umbilical vein (arrow) and two umbilical arteries (dotted arrows) are seen as a rail track appearance.

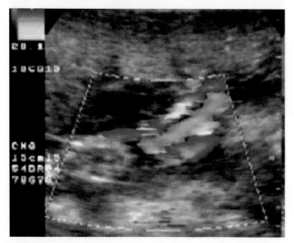

Fig. 5.179: Three vessel cord as seen on color flow mapping. Two umbilical arteries (blue) and single umbilical vein (red) can be easily demonstrated. On color flow mapping the red and blue to not specify arteries and veins but flow towards the transducer or away from it.

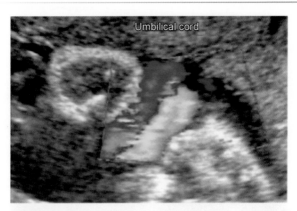

Fig. 5.180: Two vessel cord as seen on color flow mapping. Single umbilical artery and single umbilical vein can be seen.

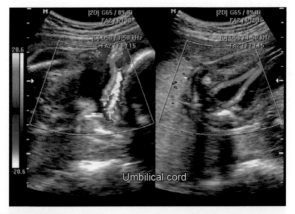

Fig. 5.181: Hypogastric arteries seen adjacent to the urinary bladder on both sides confirming a three vessel cord.

- Cervix (Internal os width, Length of cervix and Serial evaluation) (Figs. 5.183 to 5.185)
- Lower segment (Thickness)

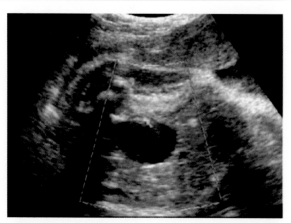

Fig. 5.182: Hypogastric artery seen adjacent to the urinary bladder only on one side confirming a two vessel cord seen in Figure 5.181.

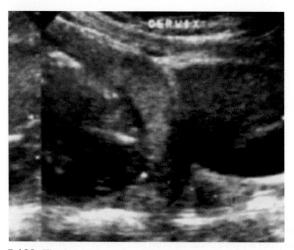

Fig. 5.183: The internal os should be seen whether it is open or not and whether there is any herniation as well.

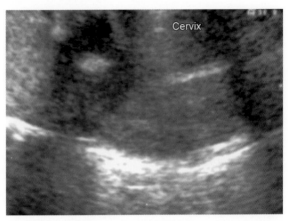

Fig. 5.184: Length: The cervical length is measured from the internal os to the external os or the mucus plug is measured.

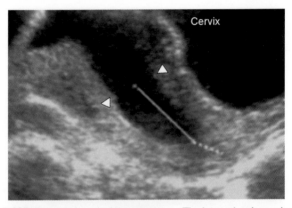

Fig. 5.185: Patient of cervical incompetence. The internal os (arrow heads) is open and 18 mm wide. The herniation of the amnion in the cervical canal (line) is over a distance of 32 mm. The functional or closed cervix (dashed line) which is required for the cerclage is 13 mm long.

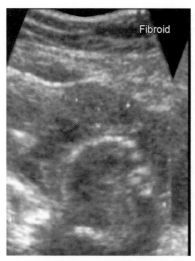

Fig. 5.186: An anterior wall subserous fibroid in a 16 weeks pregnancy.

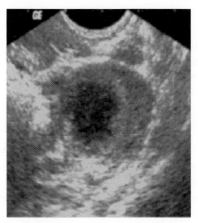

Fig. 5.187: Persistent corpus luteum in a 19 weeks pregnancy.

- Myometrium (Masses) (Fig. 5.186)
- Adnexa (Masses) (Fig. 5.187).

5.14 COLOR DOPPLER IN SECOND TRIMESTER

- Uterine artery
- Umbilical artery
- Fetal circulation
- Placental perfusion.

5.15 3D AND 4D SCAN

- Surface anatomy
- Anomaly scan
- Bone and spine evaluation
- 4D scan for maternal-fetal and family-fetal bonding.

5.16 ABNORMAL SECOND TRIMESTER

- Low placenta
- Separation
- Oligopolyhydramnios
- Single umbilical artery
- Incompetent os
- Short cervix
- Malformations.

5.17 DILEMMAS

- Is it that with ultrasound one can find out each and every problem with the fetus, color Doppler is even better and is 3D the ultimate?
- Which period is best for diagnosing anomalies?
- Is the baby low?
- Will water drinking help for making of liquor?
- Ultrasound done at 13 weeks was normal, let'us skip this scan.

Third Trimester

6.1 INDICATION

- Suspected abruptio placentae
- Estimation of fetal weight and/or presentation in premature rupture of membranes and/or premature labor
- Serial evaluation of fetal growth in multiple gestations
- Estimation of gestational age in late registrants for prenatal care
- Biophysical profile for fetal well-being
- Determination of fetal presentation
- Suspected fetal death
- Observation of intrapartum events
- Suspected polyhydramnios or oligohydramnios.

6.2 FETAL EVALUATION

- *Presentation:* Cephalic/breech (extended or footling)/oblique (Cranium in iliac fossae or hypochondrium (Figs. 6.1 and 6.2).

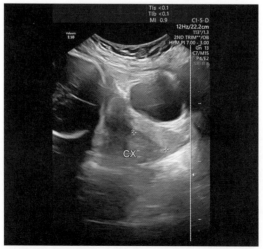

Fig. 6.1: Cephalic presentation with the cranium opposed to the cervix.

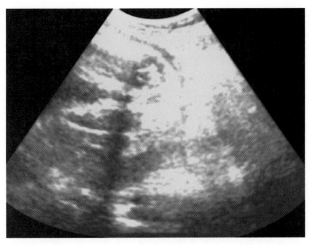

Fig. 6.2: Extended breech presentation with the fetal buttocks opposed to the cervix.

- Movements and biophysical score
- Viability
- *Gestational age:* Denotes fetal maturity (Fig. 6.3).
- *Biometry:* Denotes fetal size and weight (Figs. 6.4 to 6.6)
- Color Doppler for fetal wellbeing

6.3 EXTRA-FETAL EVALUATION

- *Placenta:* Grade I/II (with basal stippling)/III (with calcification) (Figs. 6.7 and 6.8)
- *Liquor amnii:* Normal/oligohydramnios/poly-hydramnios (Figs. 6.9 to 6.11)
- *Umbilical cord:* Presenting/around neck (Figs. 6.12 to 6.14)
- *Cervix:* Effaced/uneffaced
- *Lower segment:* Thick (normorange)/thinned (Fig. 6.15)
- Myometrium
- Adnexa.

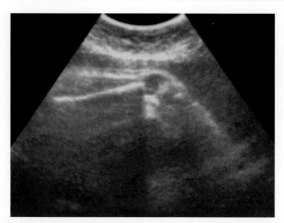

Fig. 6.3: The distal femoral epiphysis can be measured and maturity known as it starts appearing only after 35 weeks.

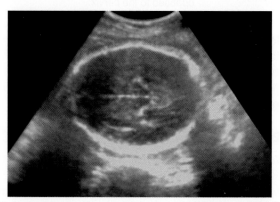

Fig. 6.4: Section for cranial biometry consisting of the thalamus, the third ventricle and the cavum septum pellucidum. The biparietal diameter is the side to side measurement from the outer table of the proximal skull to the inner table of the distal skull. The head perimeter is the total cranial circumference, which includes the maximum anteroposterior diameter. The occipito-frontal diameter is the front to back measurement from the outer table on both sides.

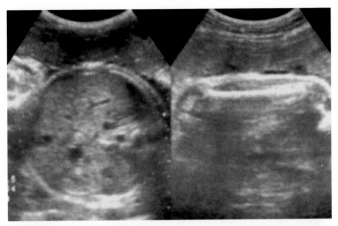

Fig. 6.5: Section for abdominal perimeter measurement. The spine should be posterior and the umbilical part of the portal vein anteriorly. Femoral length measurement for assessing fetal biometry.

```
LMP(OPE)23/11/02 GA(LMP)34W0D EDD(LMP)30/08/03    68 FO HG 20
R=f MD:                      NOTE:
         POS:                PLAC:                      + 1/2 ◘
MEASUREMENTS CUA   LAST        1      2    3      AGE        GP
BPD(HADLOCK)   u   84.6mm  (  84.6              ) 34W0D±3W1D 50%
HC(HADLOCK)    u   309mm   (  309               ) 34W4D±3W0D 26%
OFD(HC)            112mm   (  112               )
AC(HADLOCK)    u   296mm   (  296               ) 33W4D±3W0D 40%
FL(HADLOCK)    u   67.4mm  (  67.4              ) 34W5D±3W0D 50%
CRL(HADLOCK)   u           (              o     )
GS(HELLMAN)    u           (                    )




  CALCULATIONS
CI        75.7(70-86)          EFW 2328g±349g ( 5lb  2oz)   44%
FL/BPD    79.7(71-97)          Based On:(BPD HC AC  FL        )
FL/AC     22.8(20-24)            AFI(cm)       HR(BPM)
FL/HC     21.8(19.4-21.8)     LMP:(OPE)23/11/02
HC/AC     1.046(0.95-1.11)    AGE: LMP 34W0D        CUA 34W0D
                              EDD: LMP 30/08/03     CUA 30/08/03
COMMENTS:
```

Fig. 6.6: The chart shows a fetal weight of 2328 grams for 34 weeks with an EDD of 30/08/03.

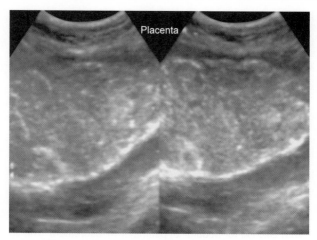

Fig. 6.7: Grade II placenta with basal stippling.

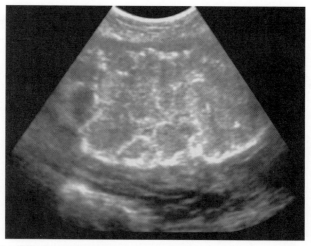

Fig. 6.8: Grade III placenta with calcification along the basal plate, chorionic plate and intercotyledons.

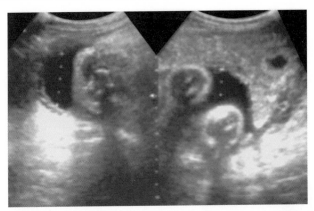

Fig. 6.9: Amniotic fluid index assessment. The uterus is divided into four quadrants by the midline and transverse axis and the amniotic fluid as the deepest vertical pocket free of fetal parts and umbilical cord is measured in each quadrant and all four quadrants add up to give the amniotic fluid index. Pregnancy of 38 weeks and 5 days with normal liquor amnii.

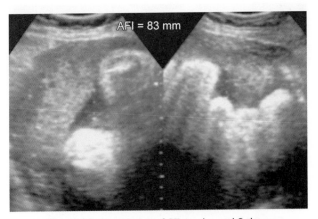

Fig. 6.10: Pregnancy of 37 weeks and 2 days with oligohydramnios.

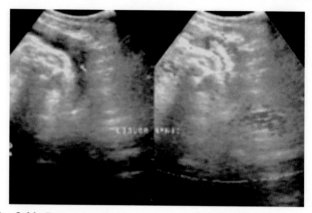

Fig. 6.11: Remember that if you have a color Doppler switch on the color to measure the pocket of liquor because many a times there is only cord in that pocket and it will give a wrong amniotic fluid index. Pocket which is full of umbilical cord so this pocket measurement is 0 mm not 28 mm as originally thought on a 2D image.

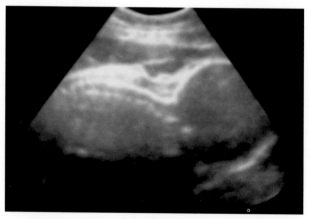

Fig. 6.12: Strong suspicion of two loops of umbilical cord on a 2D image.

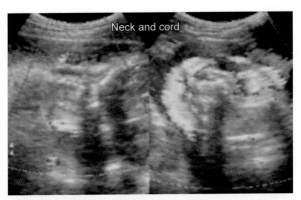

Fig. 6.13: Findings of 2D confirmed by color flow mapping when these two loops are demonstrated.

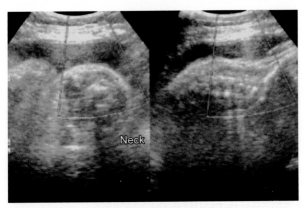

Fig. 6.14: No cord seen near or around the fetal neck as seen on color flow mapping.

6.4 PLACENTAL CHECKLIST

- Site of placentation
- Relation of lower pole to internal os < 3 cm placenta previa >3 cm-5 low lying >5 cm away normal placentation site

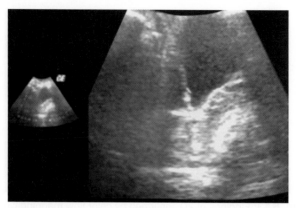

Fig. 6.15: Thinned lower segment scar seen in a patient of previous cesarean.

- Grading for maturity (immature, mature or hypermature) only hypermature placenta before 34 weeks gestation is of significance
- Check for hypoechoic space in between placenta and uterine wall (rules out placenta acreta)
- Check for retroplacental clot, abruptions, intra-placental hematomas, calcification
- Color flow imaging (angio) for number of placental vessels and vasculature (to rule out placental insufficiency and infarct).

6.5 AMNIOTIC FLUID ASSESSMENT

Condition	Single pocket	AFI
Oligohydramnios	<2 cm	<7
Reduced	2–3 cm	7–10
Normal	3–8 cm	10–17
More than average	>8–12	17–25
Polyhydramnios	>12	>25

Scan whole uterine cavity for single pocket measure largest vertical pool for AFI four quadrant method.

6.6 CAUSES OF OLIGOHYDRAMNIOS

- Idiopathic
- Decreased urine production because of bilateral renal disease (primarily renal/secondary renal dysfunction)
- Post-compensatory sequelae of intrauterine growth retardation
- Rupture of membranes
- Postmaturity

6.7 CAUSES OF POLYHYDRAMNIOS

- Idiopathic
- Open neural tube defects, e.g. encephalocele, meningomyelocele, anencephaly
- Abnormalities primarily due to gastrointestinal obstruction, e.g. esophageal atresia, duodenal atresia, small bowel atresia/obstruction or secondarily due to compression of the gastrointestinal system, e.g. cystic adenomatoid malformation, mass in the mediastinum, diaphragmatic hernia commonly left side
- Maternal diabetes mellitus
- Fetal hydrops (immune or nonimmune)
- Chromosomal abnormality: Trisomy 18.

6.8 FETAL GROWTH

Fetal growth scan influenced by:
- Small
- Large

- PIH
- APH
- Medical disorder in pregnancy
- PROM
- History of previous small births

IUGR/FGR

Causes

- Low growth potential (Intrinsic factors)
  - Genetic predisposition
  - Chromosomal anomaly
  - Fetal infection
  - Structural fetal defects
  - Drugs and medications.
- Loss of growth support (Extrinsic factors)
  - Unknown cause
  - PIH
  - Diabetes
  - Lupus
  - Recurrent bleeding episodes
  - Multiple pregnancy
  - Malnutrition
  - Drug abuse
  - Uterine anomalies

Points to Remember

- Abdominal circumference is most sensitive in 3rd trimester
- Fetal weight estimation always carries an error of ± 200 g
- Macrosomia is associated with polyhydramnios
- Shoulder dystocia in labor cannot be predicted
- Asymmetrical and symmetrical growth restriction can occur together.

6.9 FETAL SURVEILLANCE OR FETAL WELLBEING

When to evaluate:
- Unexplained fetal death
- Decreased fetal movements
- Maternal chronic hypertension
- Preeclampsia (PIH)
- Maternal diabetes mellitus
- Chronic renal disease
- Cyanotic heart disease
- Rh or other isoimmunization
- Hemoglobinopathies
- Immunological disorders
- Oligohydramnios
- Polyhydramnios
- Intrauterine growth retardation
- Multiple gestations
- Post-dated pregnancy
- Preterm labor
- Premature rupture of membranes
- History bleeding in first trimester
- Elderly women
- ART pregnancies.

6.10 BIOPHYSICAL PROFILE (FIG. 6.16)

- The fetal biophysical profile is a combination of acute and chronic markers.
- The fetal heart rate reactivity (NST), breathing movements, movements and tone are acute markers and are altered by acute hypoxic changes.
- The chronic marker of fetal condition, amniotic fluid is an indicator of chronic fetal distress and is associated with reduction of fetal cardiac output away from non-vital organs.

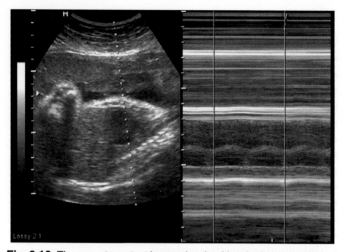

Fig. 6.16: The non-stress test is seen by checking the heart rate before and after fetal movements, to see whether there is any increase for a sufficient period of time or not.

6.11 EVALUATION BY BIOPHYSICAL PROFILE

- *Fetal breathing:* Movement is defined as 30 seconds of sustained breathing movement during a 30-minute observation period.
- *Fetal movement:* Three or more gross body movements in a 30 minute observation period
- *Fetal tone:* One or more episodes of limb motion from a position of flexion to extension and a rapid return to flexion.
- *Fetal reactivity:* Two or more FHR accelerations associated with fetal movement of at least 15 bpm and lasting at least 15 seconds in 20 minutes.
- *Fluid volume:* Presence of a pocket of amniotic fluid that measures at least 1 cm in two perpendicular planes.

6.12 INTERPRETATION OF BIOPHYSICAL PROFILE

Manning score: Each variable is allotted a score of 0–2.

- A score of >8 is normal.
- A score of 6–8 is suboptimal
- A score of <6 needs intervention.

The Manning's biophysical profile scoring is a time consuming test (at least 40 minutes). Also it takes into account four acute variables and one chronic variable. Sometimes the acute variables are affected late and remain normal (Score 8/10) while the fetus may be having severe chronic distress (AFI <5). This makes the Manning's score unpredictable. To avoid this confusion a modified score has been proposed by Vintzelo's which takes only two variables into account.

1. Liquor amnii
2. Fetal NST in response to acoustic stimulation (VAST).

This not only shortens the test duration (< 20 mins) but also makes interpretation easy and more accurate.

Interpretation

- AFI < 5. Distress delivery if viable (>28 weeks)
- If both normal wait for one week
- *If NST normal but liquor less:* Detailed color Doppler
- *If liquor normal but NST abnormal:* Acute distress
- *If both abnormal:* Individualize treatment according to gestational age.

6.13 SERIAL EVALUATION

- It is recommended that an NST be performed twice a week on all postdated, diabetic, and IUGR patients.
- Patient management is often dictated by the amount of amniotic fluid (postdate and IUGR patients). The detection of fetal anomalies combined with the ability to evaluate the amount of amniotic fluid are frequently stated as advantages of the biophysical profile over additional FHR testing in the form of OCT/CST.

6.14 COLOR DOPPLER

These are done to detect and assess the fetus at risk for death or damage in utero. Color Doppler in conjunction with 2D ultrasound and biophysical scoring is now regarded as an indispensable component of a pregnancy sonogram.

6.15 INDICATIONS FOR COLOR DOPPLER

- Assessment and continued monitoring of the small for gestational age fetus
- Assessment of the fetus of a mother with systemic lupus erythematous (SLE) and PET
- Assessment of differing sizes or growth patterns in twins
- Conjunction with uteroplacental waveforms in the assessment of oligohydramnios.

6.16 INTERPRETATION OF THE WAVEFORMS (FIGS. 6.17 TO 6.30)

- In the absence of an acute incident such as a placental abruption, a small for gestational age fetus with normal umbilical artery waveforms will not develop loss of end-diastolic frequencies within a 7-day period, so that monitoring may be performed weekly.
- Only 10% of fetuses that are demonstrated to be asymmetrically small for gestational age on real-time ultrasound will demonstrate loss of end-diastolic frequencies at any time during their pregnancy.
- Loss of end-diastolic frequencies is associated with an 85% chance that the fetus will be hypoxic *in utero* and a 50% chance that it will also be acidotic.
- The finding of a symmetrically small fetus with absent end-diastolic frequencies in the umbilical artery but with normal uteroplacental waveforms suggest the possibility of a primary fetal cause for the growth retardation such as chromosomal abnormality or a TORCH virus infection.

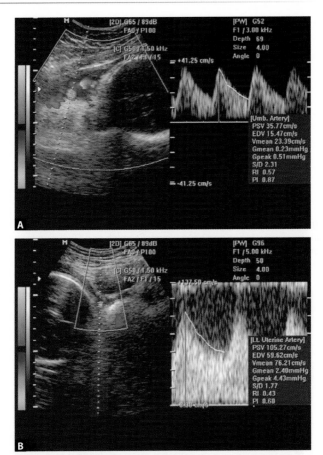

Figs. 6.17A and B: Uterine arteries reflect trophoblastic invasion and the prediction of a hypertensive disorder in low-risk mothers and perinatal morbidity and mortality in high-risk mothers. Normal uterine artery flow with flow in diastole and a resistive Index of less than 0.55 after 22 weeks (Measure the resistive indices in the (A) right and (B) left uterine arteries).

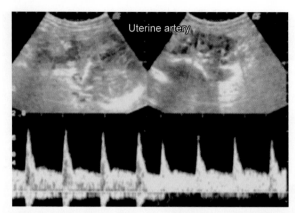

Fig. 6.18: Abnormal waveform showing a notch in early diastole. Other abnormal waveforms can have a systolic notch or a Resistive Index of more than 0.55 or a major right to left variation.

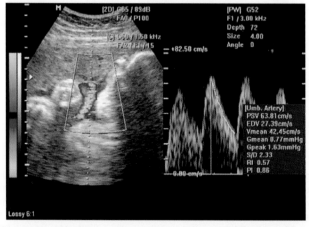

Fig. 6.19: Umbilical arteries reflect placental obliteration and one should have sufficient flow in diastole for a normal waveform.

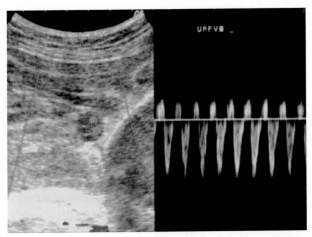

Fig. 6.20: Abnormal waveform has absent end diastolic flow or reversal of end diastolic flow. This waveform shows reversal of flow in diastole.

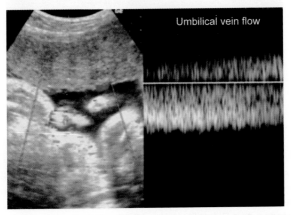

Fig. 6.21: Normal continuous flow in a umbilical vein flow pattern and this reflects myocardial function.

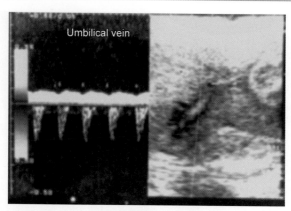

Fig. 6.22: Double pulsatile pattern seen in an abnormal umbilical vein flow pattern.

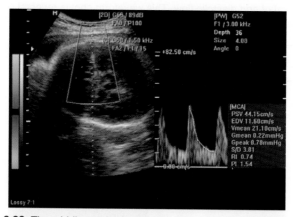

Fig. 6.23: The middle cerebral artery waveform reflects altered cerebral flow or cerebral edema. In hypoxia the blood flow to the middle cerebral artery increases as a reflex redistribution of fetal cardiac output. Normal waveform with a Pulsatility Index of 2.15.

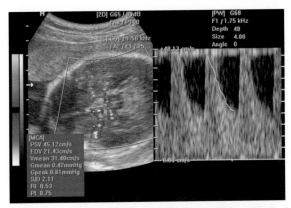

Fig. 6.24: Abnormal waveform with increased blood flow to the middle cerebral artery with a PI of 0.76.

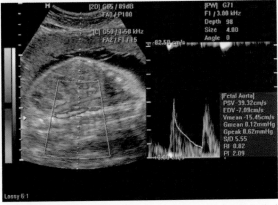

Fig. 6.25: Descending aorta reflects flow from the abdominal viscera and lower limbs. Normal waveform with adequate diastolic flow.

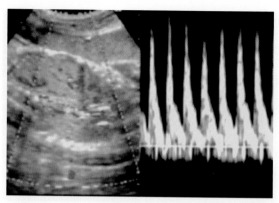

Fig. 6.26: Abnormal waveform with reduced flow in diastole for redistribution to other vital organs.

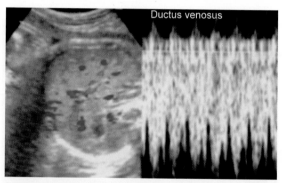

Fig. 6.27: Ductus venosus flow reflects acidosis. Normal waveform with plenty of flow in diastole.

- Fetuses demonstrating absence of end-diastolic frequencies but which are managed along standard clinical lines have a 40% chance of dying and at least a 25% morbidity rate from necrotizing enterocolitis, hemorrhage or coagulation failure after birth. The time between loss of end-diastolic

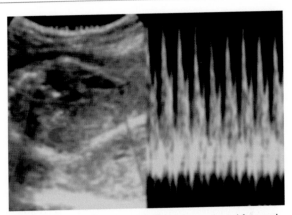

Fig. 6.28: Abnormal waveform with a reduced forward flow in diastole.

Inferior vena cava

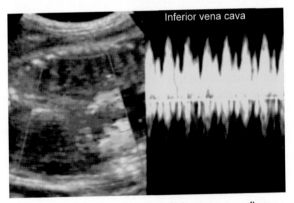

Fig. 6.29: Normal triphasic inferior vena cava flow reflecting myocardial function.

frequencies and fetal death appears to differ for each fetus, following loss of end-diastolic frequencies there are no other reliable changes in the waveform that help in deciding when to deliver the baby.

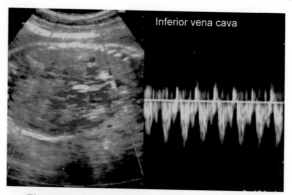

Fig. 6.30: Abnormal waveform with an increased reversed flow in diastole.

- Reversed frequencies in end-diastolic are only observed in a few fetuses prior to death. This finding is a pre-terminal condition; few if any, fetuses will service without some form of therapeutic intervention.
- Loss of end-diastolic frequencies precedes changes in the cardiotocograph by some 7–42 days in fetuses that have been shown to be small for gestational age on real-time ultrasound. The occurrence of CTG decelerations not related to contractions, together with absent end-diastolic frequencies, carries an extremely poor prognosis.
- In case of IUGR Wladimiroff and colleagues (1986) have described compensatory reduction in vascular resistance in fetal brain during fetal hypoxemia usually called as "Brain sparing effect" and is the earliest Doppler based marker for IUGR compromised fetus.
- Detection of elevated resistance to flow within fetal descending aorta reflects the decreased vascular resistance associated with high-risk pregnancy not only within the placental vascular bed but also within fetal abdominal viscera.

- Increased resistance in fetal renal arteries with growth retardation has been seen especially with oligohydramnios.
- Increased resistance in uterine artery as indicated by an elevated index of resistance by persistence of an early diastolic notch often precedes the onset of growth retardation.
- The details of normal and abnormal waveforms with their representations and end points and management protocols is discussed in detail in the Step by Step series on Ultrasound and Color Doppler.

6.17 INDICATIONS OF DELIVERY

- Viable fetus AFI < 5
- Absent end-diastolic flow or reversed end-diastolic flow in umbilical artery after 35 weeks
- Abnormal ductus venosus flow >35 weeks
- Abnormal biophysical profile.

6.18 MODE OF DELIVERY

Vaginal or cesarean section depends on cervical score, pelvis and/or any other obstetric indication for cesarean section.

6.19 ABNORMAL THIRD TRIMESTER

- Placental aging
- Separation
- Oligo/polyhydramnios
- Cord around neck
- Thinned lower segment
- Abnormal presentation
- IUGR
- Abnormal biophysical score
- Abnormal color Doppler studies.

6.20 CHECKLIST

- Calculate gestation from LMP (keep card with you)
- Fundal height clinical size
- Presentation and lie
- BPD
- HC
- AC
- FL
- Other limbs
- Head circumference
- Charts and assess growth.

6.21 DILEMMAS

- Will the ultrasound tell us the exact date of delivery
- All parameters give different EDD
- Has the internal os opened
- There is loop of cord around the neck: is it dangerous
- Has the baby come in the final position
- How many movements are normal
- First ultrasound: Please check for anomalies
- Can we wait more.

6.22 SONOGRAPHIC DIAGNOSIS OF IUGR

Disturbances of normal fetal growth can result in abnormal weight, body mass, or body proportions at birth. The two principal fetal growth disorders are intrauterine growth restriction (IUGR) and macrosomia, both associated with increased perinatal morbidity and mortality.

Intrauterine Growth Restriction

Intrauterine growth restriction is currently characterized as a syndrome marked by failure to reach growth potential.

There are several causes of IUGR. These may be conceptually divided into three main categories: maternal, fetal, and uteroplacental. It should be stressed, however, that in almost half the cases of IUGR, the etiology is unknown. IUGR has been defined variously as an infant whose birthweight is below the 3rd, 5th, and 10th percentiles for gestational age or whose birthweight is more than two standard deviations below the mean for gestational age.

Types

- Type 1 or symmetric IUGR refers to the infant with decreased growth potential. This type of IUGR begins early in gestation, and the entire fetus is proportionally SGA. Type 1 IUGR is a result of growth inhibition early in gestation, i.e. 4 to 20 weeks.
- Type 2 or asymmetric IUGR refers to the neonate with restricted growth and is most frequently due to uteroplacental insufficiency. Type 2 IUGR is a result of a later growth insult than type 1 and usually occurs after 28 weeks' gestation.
- Intermediate IUGR refers to growth restriction that is a combination of types 1 and 2 IUGR. The insult to fetal growth in intermediate IUGR most probably occurs during the middle phase of fetal growth—that of hyperplasia and hypertrophy which corresponds to 20–28 weeks gestation.[1,2]

Diagnosis

The ponderal index may identify a neonate who has a small amount of soft tissue clinically evident by loss of subcutaneous tissue and muscle mass, even though the birthweight is normal for gestational age. Neonates with a ponderal index below the 10th percentile for gestational age are probably suffering from malnutrition in utero.

Ponderal index = [birth weight (g) × 100]/[crown-heel length (cm)].[3]

6.23 ULTRASONIC MEASUREMENTS USED IN THE DIAGNOSIS OF IUGR

Ultrasound criteria have emerged as the diagnostic standard used in the identification of fetal growth restriction. Wilcocks et al. in 1964 first demonstrated the correlation between ultrasound measurement of the fetal head and birth weight. Campbell and Dewhurst published the first sonographic descriptions of fetal growth restriction with their analysis of the changes in biparietal diameter over time.

Biparietal Diameter

Biparietal diameter (BPD) was the first ultrasonic parameter used for detection of IUGR. Nomograms of BPD or head circumference (HC) are available to provide calculated estimates of weekly increments for the size of the fetal head. Hence, when comparing the observed increase in BPD with the expected rate of growth, the physician should be able to identify growth-restricted fetuses when the head is affected in the growth curtailment.

Biparietal diameter alone cannot be used as a good predictor of IUGR. Almost two-thirds of IUGR cases are of the asymmetric or late-flattening type, which have normal growth of the head until late in pregnancy as a consequence of the brain-sparing process. Therefore, BPD in asymmetric IUGR may be normal until late in gestation. Another reason for the low sensitivity of BPD measurements in detecting IUGR is the distortion of the fetal head shape that may occur, for example in dolichocephaly, or may be seen in cases of breech presentation when the BPD may be falsely small. BPD determinations, when used singly, fail to identify approximately 20–50% of IUGR infants and, therefore, cannot be used as the only parameter in screening for IUGR.

Transverse Cerebellar Diameter

The cerebellum can be easily visualized as early as the first trimester as a butterfly-shaped figure in the posterior fossa of the fetal head, behind the thalami and in front of the echolucent area (cisterna magna). The transverse cerebellar diameter (TCD) in millimeters has been shown to correlate with gestational age in weeks up to 24 weeks. TCD measurement was not significantly affected by restricted fetal growth and, therefore, the TCD could be used as a reliable predictor of gestational age even in cases of IUGR. This parameter is particularly useful because it is a standard against which other parameters can be compared. Majority of data available suggest that the use of the TCD when gestational age is unknown or IUGR is suspected is extremely valuable. The accuracy of the TCD can be enhanced by using biometric ratios, especially FL: AC, as well as amniotic fluid volume and the presence or absence of fetal ossification centres.

Abdominal Circumference

The abdominal circumference (AC) has been reported to be the best fetal biometric parameter that correlates with fetal weight and is the most sensitive parameter for detecting IUGR. In contrast to the BPD measurement, AC is smaller in both symmetric and asymmetric types of IUGR, and therefore its measurement has a higher sensitivity. Animal studies have shown that the liver is the most affected organ in IUGR. Because the liver is the largest intra-abdominal organ, assessment of the AC at the level of the liver is actually an indirect indication of the nutritional status of the fetus.

Unfortunately, AC has more intraobserver and inter-observer variation than either BPD or femur length (FL). Furthermore, AC variability may result from fetal breathing movements, compression, or position of the fetus. To obtain the proper AC, the section should be round and at the level of the fetal stomach and the portal umbilical vein (or the bifurcation of the main portal vein into the right and left branches).

Long Bones

The femur length is another important parameter in evaluating fetal growth. Long bones other than the femur can be equally useful in the assessment of gestational age. These long bones are generally decreased in symmetrically growth-restricted fetuses, but may be of normal length in asymmetric IUGR. The fetal head and long bone length in asymmetric IUGR tend to be affected late in gestation. Because the measurement of most long bones is relatively simple, they become a useful means of estimating gestational age on a routine basis.

Total Intrauterine Volume

The rationale for measuring total intrauterine volume derives from the fact that, in IUGR, intrauterine content is reduced (fetal, placental mass, and the amount of amniotic fluid). This method has been abandoned by most centers because of the widespread use of real-time ultrasonography and the fact that a static scanner is needed to measure total intrauterine volume.

Amniotic Fluid Volume Assessment

In the growth-restricted fetus, decreased amounts of amniotic fluids may be observed. This is a direct result of decreased renal perfusion and reduced urine production. Unfortunately, progressive growth curtailment usually occurs without evidence of significant amniotic fluid reduction. Hence, this parameter is not very sensitive to diagnose IUGR.

Placental Growth

Grannum and colleagues were the first to present an ultrasonic classification of placental maturity. This classification grades placentas from 0 to 3 according to specific ultrasonic findings at the basal and chronic plates, as well as within substances of the organ itself. It is noteworthy that placentas do not all necessarily go through the full maturation process during pregnancy. It has been assumed that the appearance of a grade 3 placenta before 35 weeks gestation should alert the physician to the possibility of the presence or subsequent development of IUGR. However, there are still no substantial data to support this assumption.

Body Proportionality

Indices of body proportionality that have been studied and found clinically useful include the HC/AC ratio and the FL/AC ratio.

Head circumference (HC)/abdominal circumference (AC) ratio—The rationale for this was based on the observation that type 2 IUGR may have a disturbed HC/ AC ratio as a result of the brain-sparing effect. Although this method has been shown to have a sensitivity of approximately 70% in detecting asymmetric IUGR, its use is limited by its high false-positive rate in screening a general population. Further limitations of this technique are its inability to detect asymmetric growth restriction and the need for accurate knowledge of gestational age to make the diagnosis of IUGR. It is therefore believed that the value of the HC/AC ratio lies in the assessment of proportionality, and thus it may assist the clinician in classifying IUGR as symmetric or asymmetric. An elevated ratio suggests symmetric IUGR.

Femur length (FL)/abdominal circumference (AC) ratio— The ratio of FL to AC is the equivalent of the postnatal ponderal index and has been proposed as a useful method of detecting asymmetric IUGR. This ratio has the advantage of being age independent and thus may help in the diagnosis of IUGR when gestational age is unknown. In fact, FL/AC ratios have a constant value of 22 ± 2% after 21 weeks gestation.

Estimated Fetal Weight

Several formulas that use multiple ultrasonic parameters are used to estimate fetal weight. The most widely used formula is that of Shepard and colleagues, in which estimated fetal weight (EFW) is derived from the BPD and AC. This equation predicts fetal weight with an accuracy of 15–20%. Hadlock and colleagues and Warsof and colleagues have also introduced equations to estimate fetal weight using combinations of BPD, AC, and FL. Various ultrasound methods are used to estimate fetal weight with essentially equal accuracy when low-risk obstetric populations are studied. It is thought that as many as 80% of IUGR fetuses can be detected; however, there is still a relatively low positive predictive value that approaches only 40%. Therefore, 60% of fetuses suspected of IUGR because of low EFW will actually be normally grown.

Doppler in IUGR

Maternal arterial uterine blood flow increases from 50 mL/min early in pregnancy to about 700 mL/min at term. The increase is secondary to a gradual decrease in vessel resistance to blood flow throughout the pregnancy. Doppler ultrasound gives us information on the vascular resistance and, indirectly, on the blood flow.

Three indices are considered to be related to the vascular resistance: S/D ratio (systolic/diastolic ratio), resistance index (RI = systolic velocity–diastolic velocity/systolic velocity), and pulsatility index (systolic velocity–diastolic velocity/ mean velocity). Doppler velocimetry uses ultrasound to measure peak-systolic and end-diastolic blood flow through the umbilical artery.

As the pregnancy progresses, diastolic flow increases, and the systolic/diastolic ratio should gradually decrease. In a large number of IUGR pregnancies, an alteration in placental blood flow occurs. As a result, researchers have correlated an increased systolic/diastolic ratio with IUGR. The ratio is increased in about 80% of cases of IUGR diagnosed by ultrasound examination. An average systolic/diastolic ratio of greater than three at 30 or more weeks of gestation has a sensitivity of 78% and a specificity of 85% in predicting IUGR.

Uterine Circulation

The main uterine artery is the most commonly analyzed vessel. In normal pregnancy, the S/D ratio or RI values decrease significantly with advancing gestation until 24–26 weeks. In the absence of this physiologic decrease, a higher incidence of hypertensive diseases and/or IUGR has been widely documented.

Umbilical Artery

The common method used to evaluate umbilical artery wave form is to pick any free-floating loop of cord, usually with color Doppler, and to obtain the waveform from it with pulsed Doppler. In the normal fetus, the pulsatility index decreases with advancing gestation. This reflects a decrease in the placental vascular resistance. In fetuses with IUGR, there is an increase in the pulsatility index secondary to the decrease, absence, or reversal of end-diastolic flow. The changes in these waveforms are thought to be indicative of increased placental resistance. The absent or reversed end-diastolic flows are strongly associated with an abnormal course of pregnancy and a higher incidence of perinatal complications.

Fetal Cerebral Circulation

The middle cerebral artery is the vessel of choice to assess the fetal cerebral circulation because it is easy to identify, has a high reproducibility, and provides information on the brain sparing effect. The circulation in the brain is normally high impedance. The middle cerebral artery (MCA) in the fetal brain carries more than 80% of cerebral flow. When a fetus does not acquire enough oxygen, central redistribution of blood flow occurs, resulting in a preferentially increased blood flow to protect the brain, heart, and adrenals. This increase in blood flow can be evidenced by Doppler ultrasound of the MCA. This effect has been called the brain-sparing effect and is demonstrated by a lower value of the pulsatility index.

In IUGR fetuses with a pulsatility index below the normal range, there is a greater incidence of adverse perinatal outcome. The brain-sparing effect may be transient, as reported during prolonged hypoxemia. The disappearance of the brain-sparing effect is a very critical event for the fetus, and appears to precede fetal death.

Fetal Venous Doppler

Doppler flow of the fetal inferior vena cava (IVC) and ductus venosus is practical and provides information about right ventricle preload, myocardial compliance, and right ventricular end-diastolic pressure. Chronic fetal hypoxemia leads to decreased preload, decreased cardiac compliance, and elevated end-diastolic pressure in the right ventricle. These changes raise central venous pressure in the chronically hypoxemic fetus, which shows up as an increased reverse flow in Doppler waveforms of the IVC and the ductus venosus during late diastole (Box 6.1). Changes in the fetal central venous circulation are associated with an advanced stage of fetal hypoxemia.

Box 6.1: Explanation of Doppler indices

A/C ratio	Ratio of peak systolic to early diastolic velocity
Any notching	Presence of early diastolic notching* in waveform; may be unilateral or bilateral
Bilateral notching	Presence of early diastolic notching in waveform of both main uterine arteries
D/S ratio	Ratio of diastolic to systolic velocity
D/S or notching	D/S ratio with or without unilateral or bilateral early diastolic notching
Notch index (or notch depth index)	Notch flow minus early diastolic flow divided by notch flow: (D–C)/D
Pulsatility index	Peak systolic flow minus end diastolic flow divided by mean flow: (A–B)/M
Pulsatility index and notching	Pulsatility index combined with unilateral or bilateral early diastolic notching
Pulsatility index or notching	Pulsatility index with or without unilateral or bilateral early diastolic notching
Resistance index	Peak systolic flow minus end diastolic flow divided by peak systolic flow: (A–B)/A
Resistance index and notching	Resistance index combined with unilateral or bilateral early diastolic notching
Resistance index or notching	Resistance index with or without unilateral or bilateral early diastolic notching
S/D ratio	Ratio of peak systolic to late diastolic velocity (also known as A/B ratio)
S/D or notching	S/D ratio with or without unilateral of bilateral early diastolic notching
Unilateral notching	Presence of early diastolic notching in waveform of one main uterine artery

*Early diastolic notching = characteristic wave form indicating decreased early diastolic flow in the uterine artery compared with later diastolic flow.

At this late stage of fetal adaptation to hypoxemia, cardiac decompensation is often noted with myocardial dysfunction. The presence of reversed flow in the ductus venosus is an

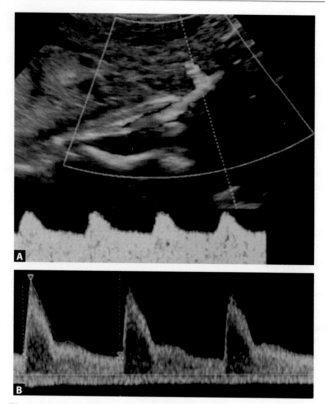

Figs. 6.31A and B: (A) Normal and (B) Abnormal uterine artery Doppler flow.

ominous sign. Indeed, fetal metabolic acidemia is often present in association with Doppler waveform abnormalities of the IVC and ductus venosus (Figs. 6.31A and B).

SUMMARY

Although the etiology of IUGR is variable, prenatal diagnosis is possible using a variety of biometric parameters. When the

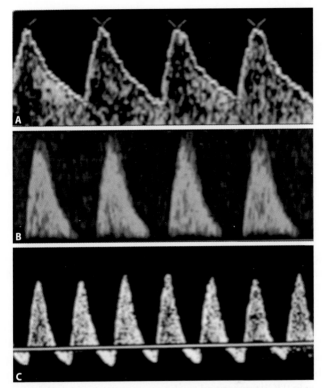

Figs. 6.32A to C: (A) Normal umbilical artery Doppler flow wave form; (B) Absent and; (C) reversed end-diastolic Doppler flow in umbilical artery.

gestational age is certain, IUGR is diagnosed if sonographic predictors of gestational age reflect an age significantly reduced from the expected, or an EFW less than the 10th percentile. Adjunctive indices that can enhance the prenatal diagnosis include reduced amniotic fluid volume, early third trimester grade 3 placenta, abnormal Doppler waveform analysis, and abnormal biometric ratios (Figs. 6.32 and 6.33).

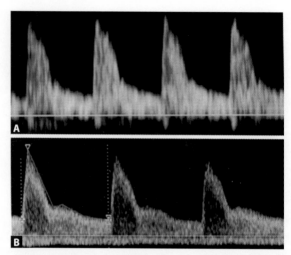

Figs. 6.33A and B: (A) Normal middle cerebral artery Doppler flow wave form; (B) Abnormal middle cerebral artery Doppler flow with increased diastolic flow (brain sparing).

When the gestational age is unknown or uncertain, it is necessary to differentiate between the IUGR fetus and the normally grown fetus identified at an inaccurate gestational age. The TCD is a useful parameter for estimating gestational age even in IUGR fetuses and can be a parameter against which other biometric indices are compared. Biometric ratios, especially FL/AC, may also be useful adjuncts in the prenatal diagnosis of IUGR.

REFERENCES

1. American College of Obstetricians and Gynecologists. Intrauterine growth restriction; ACOG practice bulletin no. 12. Washington, DC: ACOG; 2000. Level III.
2. Baschat AA. Arterial and venous Doppler in the diagnosis and management of early onset fetal growth restriction. Early Hum Dev. 2005;81:877-87. Level III.

3. Jauniaux E, Jurkovic D, Campbell S, et al. Doppler ultrasonographic features of the developing placental circulation; correlation with anatomic findings. Am J Obstet Gynecol. 1992;166:585-7. Level II-3.

4. Papageorghiou AT, Yu CKH, Nicolaides KH. The role of uterine artery Doppler in predicting adverse pregnancy outcome. Best Pract Res Clin Obstet Gynecol. 2004;18:383-96. Level III.

5. Campbell S, Diaz-Recasens J, Griffin DR, et al. New Doppler technique for assessing uteroplacental blood flow. Lancet. 1983;26:675-7. Level II-3.

6. Sciscione AC, Hayes EJ. Society for Maternal-Fetal Medicine: uterine artery Doppler flow studies in obstetric practice. Am J Obstet Gynecol. 2009;201:121-6. Level III.

6.24 COLOR DOPPLER IN IUGR

The development of a good utero-placental circulation is essential for the achievement of a normal pregnancy. Color Doppler:

- Gives information regarding circulation
- Can be used repetitively
- Noninvasive
- Can reliably predict adverse perinatal outcome in an IUGR pregnancy
- Compared to other methods of monitoring more sensitive in predicting fetal compromise early
- Helpful in deciding time of delivery.

The vessels to be studied are:

- Uterine arteries
  - They reflect uteroplacental flow
  - Normally changes from one of low peak flow velocity and early diastolic notch to one of high peak flow and no diastolic notch by 18–22 weeks
  - PI at 18–22 weeks is <1.2
  - PI >1.45 and presence of early diastolic notch in B/L uterine arteries at 18–22 weeks is s/o uteroplacental insufficiency (Figs. 6.34 and 6.35).[1]

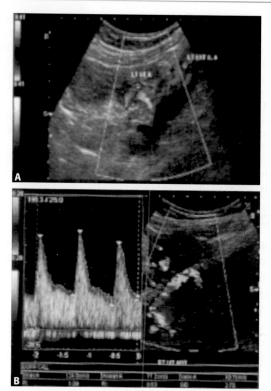

Figs. 6.34A and B: The spectral waveform of the right uterine artery shows a normal early diastolic notch which is normally seen till the age of 25 weeks of gestation. PI and RI values early in the pregnancy can be quite high signifying increased resistance in the placental and chorionic vascular beds. Thus PI values are typically higher than 2.5 in 11–14 week period, decreasing gradually as the gestation progresses. However, PI and RI values can vary depending on placental position (with low PI values in the uterine artery on the side of the placenta). Persistence of the diastolic notch and high PI and RI values can signify danger of the preeclampsia, placental abruption and PIH (pregnancy induced hypertension), and IUGR. Thus uterine artery Doppler can be used to predict or exclude danger to the fetus in the coming months. The left uterine artery in the color Doppler image above is smaller in size due to the placenta being more on the right side of the uterus.

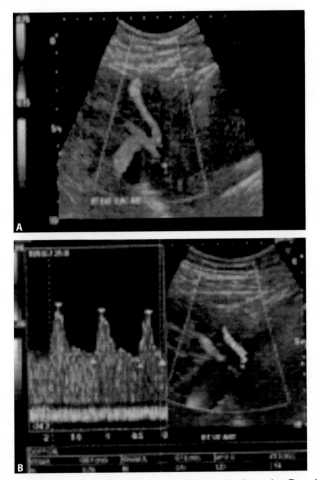

Figs. 6.35A and B: The right uterine artery in the color Doppler ultrasound image (A) shows bifurcation or division just before it crosses the right external iliac artery and vein. This was a 24-week-old pregnancy. The spectral Doppler ultrasound image on (B) shows normal low resistance flow cynically seen at this stage of pregnancy. RI of the uterine artery in this case measures 0.51, well within the normal limits.

Whenever there is any problem, earliest changes appear in umbilical and middle cerebral arteries followed by other peripheral arteries. If adequate measures are not taken at this point, venous changes appear. These are strong predictors of poor perinatal outcome and indicate impending irreversible damage.

Doppler reveals changes of hypoxia at least a week before the non-stress test or the biophysical profile. It has therefore become the gold standard in the management of growth restricted.

Umbilical Artery Doppler

It is a direct reflection of flow in placenta, **Signature vessel**.

It is the first vessel to be studied when suspecting IUGR.

UA Doppler is the only measure that provides both diagnostic and prognostic information for the management of FGR. On the one hand, increased UA Doppler PI has a great clinical value for the identification of FGR fetuses, alone or combined in the CPR ratio. Diastolic flow is seen by 14–16 weeks. PI falls from 2 to 1 as pregnancy progresses.

There is compelling evidence that using UA Doppler in high-risk pregnancies (most of them SGA fetuses) improves perinatal outcomes, with a 29% reduction (2–48%) in perinatal deaths.[2] Absent or reversed end-diastolic velocities, the end of the spectrum of the abnormalities of the UA Doppler, have been reported to be present on average one week before the acute deterioration. Up to 40% of fetuses with acidosis show this umbilical flow pattern.[3] There is an association between reversed end-diastolic flow in the UA and adverse perinatal outcome (with a sensitivity and specificity of about 60%), which seems to be independent of prematurity. After 30 weeks the risk of stillbirth of a fetus with isolated reversed end-diastolic velocities in the UA Doppler overcomes the risks of prematurity, and therefore delivery seems justified (Figs. 6.36A and B).

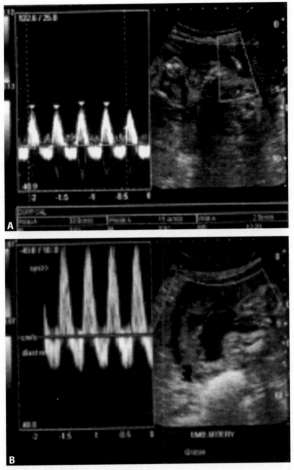

Figs. 6.36A and B: Color Doppler and spectral waveform imaging of the umbilical artery shows reversal of diastolic flow. This is an ominous sign of fetal compromise/ hypoxia and requires us to evaluate the fetal middle cerebral artery and ductus venosus. The diastolic flow reversal in umbilical arteries signifies severe placental insufficiency and increased placental vascular resistance, which is bad news for the fetus.

Middle Cerebral Artery Doppler

Vasodilation in MCA is a surrogate marker of hypoxia (Figs. 6.37A and B). MCA is considered a rather late manifestation, with acceptable specificity but low sensitivity, which is improved by the use of CPR, as discussed below. There is an association between abnormal MCA PI and adverse perinatal and neurological outcome, but it is unclear whether delivering before term could add any benefit. MCA is particularly valuable for the identification[4] and prediction[5] of adverse outcome among late-onset FGR, independently of the UA Doppler, which is often normal in these fetuses. Fetuses with abnormal MCA PI had a six fold risk of emergency cesarean section for fetal distress when compared with SGA fetuses with normal MCA PI, which is particularly relevant because labor induction at term is the current standard of care of late-onset FGR. Late FGRs with abnormal MCA PI have poorer neurobehavioral competence at birth and at 2 years of age.

Cerebroplacental Ratio

The CPR is essentially a diagnostic index. It is derived by dividing MCA PI by UA PI. The value is expressed as multiples of median (MoM). The CPR incorporates the data of both placental status (UA) and fetal response (MCA) in the prediction of adverse outcomes. It is considered abnormal below 1.08. In normal pregnancy it remains constant in last 10 weeks. The CPR improves remarkably the sensitivity of UA and MCA alone, because increased placental impedance (UA) is often combined with reduced cerebral resistance (MCA). Thus, the CPR is already decreased when its individual components suffer mild changes but are still within normal ranges.[6] In late SGA fetuses, abnormal CPR is present before delivery in 20–25% of the cases, and it is associated with a higher risk of adverse outcome at induction, although to a

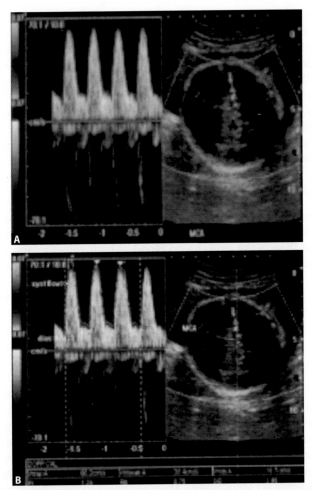

Figs. 6.37A and B: Color Doppler and spectral waveform of the middle cerebral artery shows increased diastolic flow in the fetal brain suggesting a "fetal brain sparing" effect, whereby, the fetal cerebral vessels "open up", lowering the cerebral vascular resistance to increase flow to the brain thus diverting blood to the important organs in a state of overall fetal hypoxia.

lesser degree than MCA.[7] There are no long-term studies evaluating the neurobehavioral or neurodevelopmental consequences of late SGA with abnormal CPR. However, it is remarkable that even in the general population, an abnormal CPR predicts neurobehavioral problems at 18 months of age. Interestingly, the anterior cerebral artery-CPR rather than the MCA-CPR showed the stronger association, demonstrating a differential impact of regional alterations in cerebral blood flow impedance on development, which is consistent with findings in early FGR.

Ductus Venosus Doppler

Ductus venosus is a muscularized narrow channel which receives approx. 50% of flow from intrahepatic umbilical vein and directs the oxygenated blood at high velocity (approx. 60 cm/sec) via foramen ovale into left atrium and onwards to aortic arch and fetal brain.

- Only venous channel with continuous forward flow during entire cardiac cycle
- Normal waveform shows a peak systolic, peak diastolic and a peak atrial velocity ('a' wave due to atrial contractions and smaller 'e' wave due to tricuspid valve closure)
- Normally PSV is 50 cms/sec with small 'a' wave

Ductus venosus (DV) is the strongest single Doppler parameter to predict the short-term risk of fetal death in early-onset FGR (Figs. 6.38A and B). Longitudinal studies have demonstrated that DV flow waveforms become abnormal only in advanced stages of fetal compromise.[8] Consistently, there is a good correlation of abnormal DV waveform with late-stage acidemia at cordocentesis. Absent or reversed velocities during atrial contraction are associated with perinatal mortality independently of the gestational age at delivery,[9] with a risk ranging from 40% to 100% in early-onset FGR. Thus, this sign is normally considered sufficient to recommend delivery at any gestational age, after completion of steroids. A DV above the 95% centile is associated with higher risks but not as consistently as when atrial flow is reverse. Overall, the sensitivity for perinatal death is still 40–70%.[9] A systematic review of 18 observational studies (including 2,267 fetuses) found that DV Doppler has predictive capacity for perinatal mortality. In about 50% of cases, abnormal DV precedes the loss of short-term variability (STY) in computerized cardiotocography (cCTG), and in about 90% of cases it is abnormal 48–72 h before the biophysical profile (BPP).[8] Hence, it is considered to provide a better window of opportunity for delivering fetuses in critical conditions at very early gestational ages.

Umbilical Vein (Figs. 6.38A to D)

It has continuous forward flow throughout the cycle and gradually increases from the 20th to 38th weeks. of gestation. In severe cases, when there is reversal of flow in the IVC and DV due to right heart failure, a pulsatile flow pattern begins to appear due to high resistance to forward flow. The presence of umbilical vein pulsations is associated with an increased risk of adverse perinatal outcome (Figs. 6.39A and B).

Aortic Isthmus Doppler

The aortic isthmus (AoI) Doppler is associated with increased fetal mortality and neurological morbidity in early-onset FGR.[10] This vessel reflects the balance between the impedance of the brain and systemic vascular systems. Reverse AoI flow is a sign of advanced deterioration and a further step in the sequence starting with the UA and MCA Dopplers (Figs. 6.40 and 6.41). Remarkably, the AoI can be found abnormal also in a small proportion of late-onset FGRs.

AoI has a strong association with both adverse perinatal[11] and neurological outcome.[10] However, longitudinal studies show that the AoI precedes DV abnormalities by 1 week, and

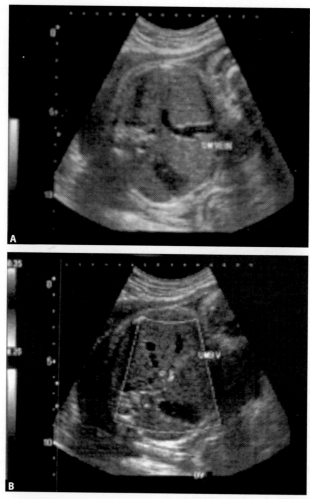

Figs. 6.38A and B: It is often difficult to snot the ductus venosus among the numerous vessels in the fetal abdomen. The easy wayout is (A) first spot the umbilical vein passing through the fetal abdomen; (B) switch on the color Doppler function to view the flow of the umbilical vein.

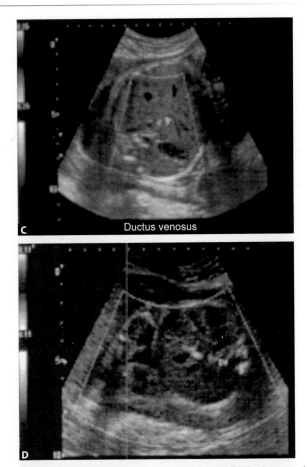

Figs. 6.38C and D: (C) Reduce or increase the PRF (pulse repetition frequency) function of the color flow until you spot a prominent but short vessel with MARKED ALIASING (i.e.: turbulent flow producing a multiple shades in the flow image). This is most likely to be the ductus venosus. Note the location of the vessel, just anterior to the fetal aorta; (D) now switch on the spectral doppler trace of the vessel. This will give a wavy spectral waveform with 3 waves: The S wave, the D wave and the A wave. Note the marked diastolic flow in this waveform. This is diagnostic of a normal Ductus venosus.

consequently it is not as good to predict the short-term risk of stillbirth. In contrast, AoI seems to improve the prediction of neurological morbidity.[10] Among early-onset FGR with positive DV atrial velocities, a reverse AoI indicated a very high risk of late neonatal neurological injury (57% vs 9.7%). In the opinion of the authors, reverse AoI could already be incorporated in clinical protocols as a sign of severe placental insufficiency and could justify considering elective delivery beyond 34 weeks of gestation. If future studies confirm the strong association with neurological morbidity, reverse AoI flow could be used to indicate delivery even earlier, but more data are required.

CONCLUSION

- Placental insufficiency is the most common cause of IUGR.
- The preventive role of uterine artery Doppler is shifting to first trimester together with biochemical markers in suspected cases.

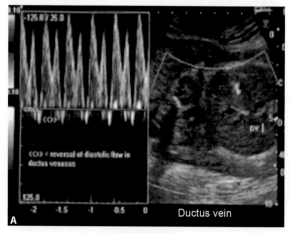

Fig. 6.39A

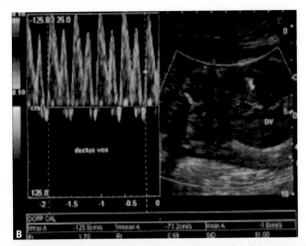

Figs. 6.39A and B: Doppler spectral waveform of the ductus venosus shows not just absent diastolic flow, but actual flow reversal during diastole. This is an ominous sign and suggest severe fetal compromise (i.e. hypoxia). It is associated with very high fetal morbidity and mortality. In this fetus, the resistance Index for the vessels in this case are as follows: Umbilical artery: 0.92; MCA: 0.75; DV: 0.99

The cerebro-placental ratio = RI (mca)/RI (umb. a.) = 0.75/0.92 = 0.81. The normal ratio is >1. This suggests severe fetal growth retardation (IUGR) in this fetus possibly due to severe placental insufficiency. Ultrasound imaging and biometry also confirmed evidence of growth retardation in this fetus (28 weeks by ultrasound versus 31 weeks by last menstrual period). All these ultrasound and color doppler images suggest fetal growth retardation with fetal compromise and anoxia—meaning we have a very sick fetus that needs prompt delivery.

- Cerebro-placental ratio, resultant of middle cerebral and umbilical arteries appears to be better parameter when in mild cases stand alone umbilical artery study is normal.
- The advent of aortic isthmus is a new ray of hope. Greater the reverse isthmic flow, higher the risk of potential cerebral damage. Aortic isthmus Doppler may prove to be a better vessel to image as compared to DV in improving

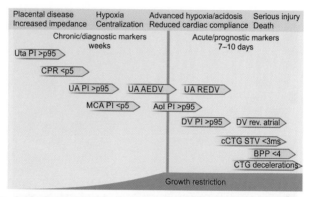

Fig. 6.40: Fetal deterioration and monitoring in early-severe FGR. Placental disease affects a large proportion of the placenta, and this is reflected in changes in the UA Doppler in a high proportion of cases. The figure depicts in a schematic and simplified fashion the pathophysiologic progression with the main adaptation/consequence in placental-fetal physiology, and the accompanying cascade of changes in Doppler parameters. The sequence illustrates the average temporal relation among changes in parameters, but the actual duration of deterioration is influenced by severity. Regardless of the velocity of progression, in the absence of accompanying PE this sequence is relatively constant, particularly as regards end-stage signs and the likelihood of serious injury/death. However, severe PE may distort the natural history and fetal deterioration may occur unexpectedly at any time.
(Uta: Uterine artery; CPR: Cerebro placental ratio; UA: Umbilical artery; MCA: Middle cerebral artery; AoI: Aortc isthmus; DV: Ductus venosus; PI: Pulsatility index; AEDV: Absent end diastolic velocity; REDV: Reverse end diastolic velocity; cCTG: Computerized cardiotocography).

long-term neuro-logical morbidity in the severely hypoxic preterm fetus.[11]

- Recent studies have documented adverse long term neurological sequelae even in those fetuses subjected to hypoxia for a short duration, hence the role of Doppler has shifted from a curative to a preventive one with truly informed and meaningful brain-oriented fetal care becoming a clinical reality.

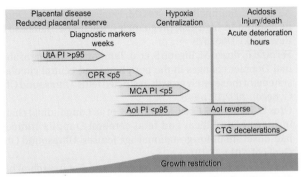

Fig. 6.41: Fetal deterioration and monitoring in late-mild FGR. Placental disease is mild and UA Doppler values are not elevated above the 95th centile. The effects of fetal adaptation are best detected by the CPR, which can pick up mild changes in the UA and MCA Doppler. An important fraction of cases do not progress to baseline hypoxia so that they remain only with abnormal CPR. Once baseline hypoxia is established, placental reserve is minimal and progression to fetal deterioration may occur quickly, as suggested by the high risk of severe deterioration or intrauterine fetal death after 37 weeks in these cases, possibly due to a combination of a higher susceptibility to hypoxia of the term-mature fetus and the more common presence of contractions at term.
(UtA: Uterine artery; CPR: Cerebro placental ratio; MCA: Middle cerebral artery; AoI: Aortc isthmus; PI: Pulsatility index; cCTG: Computerized cardiotocography).

- Regular fetal monitoring using color Doppler is helpful in prolonging pregnancy to term with reduced perinatal morbidity and mortality.
- Mild late onset IUGR must be looked for as they are a serious and substantial causes of stillbirth.

REFERENCES

1. Palma-Dias RS, Fonseca MM, Brietzke E, et al. Screening for placental insufficiency by transvaginal uterine artery Doppler at 22–24 weeks of gestation. Fetal Diagn Ther. 2008;24(4):462-9.

2. Alfirevic Z, Stampalija T, Gyte GM. Fetal and umbilical Doppler ultrasound in high-risk pregnancies. Cochrane Database Syst Rev. 2010:CD007529

3. Ferrazzi E, Bozzo M, Rigano S, et al. Temporal sequence of abnormal Doppler changes in the peripheral and central circulatory systems of the severely growth-restricted fetus. Ultrasound Obstet Gynecol. 2002;19:140-6.

4. Oros D, Figueras F, Cruz-Martinez R, et al. Longitudinal changes in uterine, umbilical and fetal cerebral Doppler indices in late-onset small-for-gestational age fetuses. Ultrasound Obstet Gynecol. 2011;37:191-5.

5. Hershkovitz R, Kingdom JC, Geary M, et al. Fetal cerebral blood flow redistribution in late gestation: identification of compromise in small fetuses with normal umbilical artery Doppler. Ultrasound Obstet Gynecol. 2000;15:209-12.

6. Gramellini D, Folli MC, Raboni S, et al. Cerebral-umbilical Doppler ratio as a predictor of adverse perinatal outcome. Obstet Gynecol. 1992;79:416-20.

7. Cruz-Martinez R, Figueras F, Hernandez-Andrade E, et al. Fetal brain Doppler to predict cesarean delivery for nonreassuring fetal status in term small-for-gestational-age fetuses. Obstet Gynecol. 2011;117:618-26.

8. Baschat AA, Gembruch U, Harman CR. The sequence of changes in Doppler and biophysical parameters as severe fetal growth restriction worsens. Ultrasound Obstet Gynecol. 2001;18:571-7.

9. Schwarze A, Gembruch U, Krapp M, et al. Qualitative venous Doppler flow waveform analysis in preterm intrauterine growth-restricted fetuses with ARED flow in the umbilical artery-correlation with short-term outcome. Ultrasound Obstet Gynecol. 2005;25:573-9.

10. Fouron JC, Gosselin J, Raboisson MJ, et al. The relationship between an aortic isthmus blood flow velocity index and the postnatal neurodevelopmental status of fetuses with placental circulatory insufficiency. Am J Obstet Gynecol. 2005;192:497-503.

11. Del Río M, Martínez JM, Figueras F, et al. Doppler assessment of the aortic isthmus and perinatal outcome in preterm fetuses with severe intrauterine growth restriction. Ultrasound Obstet Gynecol. 2008;31:41-7.

PCPNDT Act

PCPNDT (PRECONCEPTIONAL PRENATAL DIAGNOSTIC TECHNIQUES) ACT

Why This Act

An Act to provide for the prohibition of sex selection, before or after conception, and for regulation of prenatal diagnostic techniques (PNDT) for the purposes of detecting genetic abnormalities or metabolic disorders or chromosomal abnormalities or certain congenital malformations or sex-linked disorders and for the prevention of their misuse for sex determination leading to female feticide and for matters connected therewith or incidental there to.

Prenatal Diagnostic Techniques

These include:
- Prenatal diagnostic procedures
- Prenatal diagnostic tests
- Sex selection.

As per Notification in Gazette on 7.2.12 by GDR BO(E) the following were inserted in definition:
- ***"Mobile medical unit"*** *means a mobile vehicle which provides specialized facilities for the patients.*

- *"Mobile genetic clinic"* means a mobile medical unit where ultrasound machine or imaging machine is used.

Under this Act there is provision of registration in three categories as under:

- *Genetic counseling center:* The qualifications of the employees, for a Genetic Counseling Center (GCC) shall be as under rule 3 (1): A gynecologist or a pediatrician having 6 months experience or 4 weeks training in genetic counseling or a medical geneticists.

- *Genetic laboratory:* The qualifications of the employees, the requirement of equipment, etc. for a genetic laboratory (GL) shall be as under rule 3 (2): Any person having adequate space and being or employing
  - A medical geneticist
  - A laboratory technician, having a BSc degree in biological sciences or a degree or diploma in medical laboratory course with at least 1 year experience in conducting appropriate prenatal diagnostic techniques, tests or procedures.

- *Genetic clinic/ultrasound clinic/imaging center:* The qualifications of the employees, the requirement of equipment, etc. for a Genetic Clinic/Ultrasound Clinic/Imaging Center after GSR 13(E) 2014. rule 3 (3): Any person having adequate space and being or employing
  - Gynecologist having experience of performing at least 20 procedures

    or
  - A sonologist or imaging specialist or registered medical practitioner having Postgraduate degree or diploma or 6 months training duly imparted in the manner prescribed in "the Preconception and PNDT (Prohibition of Sex Selection) (6 Months Training) Rules, 2014."

or
- A medical geneticist may set up a genetic clinic/ultrasound clinic/imaging center.
- For in vitro fertilization (IVF) center there is no separate category. In IVF center, we are giving genetic counseling, prenatal diagnostic procedure and test. So registration in all three categories is sufficient for IVF center.

Amendment 2012 by Notification in Gazette on 7.2.2012

38 (1). Regulation of portable machines: The use of portable ultrasound machine or any other portable machine or device which has the potential for selection of sex before conception or detection of sex during pregnancy shall be permitted only in the following conditions, namely:
- The portable machine being used, within the premises it is registered, for providing services to the indoor patients,
- As part of a mobile medical unit, offering a bouquet of other health and medical services; explanation-for the purpose of this sub-rule, the expression "other health and medical services" means the host of services provided by the mobile medical unit.

Registration of Genetic Counseling Center, Genetic Laboratory, Ultrasound Clinic and Genetic Clinic

- An application for registration shall be made to the appropriate authority, i.e. DM/CMO in duplicate, in Form A.
- The Appropriate Authority, or any person in his office authorized in this behalf, shall acknowledge receipt of the application for registration, in the acknowledgement slip provided at the bottom of Form A, immediately if delivered at the office of the Appropriate Authority, or not later than the next working day if received by post.

As per Notification date 4.6.2012

Fee for Registration in One Category .... ₹ 25,000/

Fee for Registration in Two or Three Category .... ₹ 35,000/ for Five Year

- Renewal Fee is Half of Registration

    Ultrasound machine, sonologist and place of doing ultrasound are registered together. In case of mobile ultrasound machine, place of doing obstetric ultrasound should also be registered separately.

- Registration or Rejection

    Grant of certificate of registration or rejection of application for registration shall be communicated to the applicant as specified in Form B or Form C, as the case may be, within a period of 70 days from the date of receipt of application for registration.

Renewal of Registration

An application for renewal of certificate of registration shall be made in duplicate in Form A, to the Appropriate Authority 30 days before the date of expiry of the certificate of registration. Acknowledgement of receipt of such application shall be issued by the Appropriate Authority in the manner as for registration. In the event of failure of the Appropriate Authority to renew the certificate of registration or to communicate rejection of application for renewal of registration within a period of 70 days from the date of receipt of application for renewal of registration, the certificate of registration shall be deemed to have been renewed (GSR119 E).

Appropriate Authority and Advisory Committee— As per Rule 17

- The Central Government shall appoint, by notification in the Official Gazette, one or more Appropriate Authorities for each of the Union Territories for the purposes of this Act.

- The State Government shall appoint, by notification in the Official Gazette, one or more Appropriate Authorities for the whole or part of the State for the purposes of this Act having regard to the intensity of the problem of prenatal sex determination leading to female feticide.

District Advisory Committee

- Three medical experts from amongst gynecologists, obstetricians, pediatricians and medical geneticists
- One legal expert
- One officer to represent the department dealing with information and publicity of the State Government or the Union Territory, as the case may be.
- Three eminent social workers of whom not less than one shall be from amongst representatives of women's organizations.

Appropriate Authority

The Appropriate Authority shall have the following functions, namely:

- To grant, suspend or cancel registration of a GCC, GL or Genetic Clinic.
- To enforce standards prescribed for the GCC, GL and Genetic Clinic.
- To investigate complaints of breach of the provisions of this Act or the "rules made there under and take immediate action.
- To seek and consider the advice of the Advisory Committee, constituted under Sub-Section (5), on application for registration and on complaints for suspension or cancellation of registration.

Offences and Penalties

- Prohibition of advertisement relating to preconception and prenatal determination of sex.

- Owner of the place or any employee (permanent or honorary).
- *For first contravention*: Imprisonment up to 3 years and with fine which may extend to ₹ 10,000
- *For subsequent contravention*: Imprisonment up to 5 years and with fine which may extend up to ₹ 50,000
- The name of the Registered Medical Practitioner shall be reported by the to the State Medical Council concerned for taking necessary actions
- *Suspension of registration*: If the charges are framed by the Court and till the case is disposed-off
- Removal of the name from the register of the council:
  - For 5 Years for the first conviction
  - Permanently for subsequent offence
- Contravention of any provisions or any rules for which no penalty has been elsewhere provided in this Act, punishment is imprisonment up to 3 months or fine up to ₹ 1,000 or both.
- Continuing contravention additional ₹ 500 for every day during which such contravention continues after conviction for the first such contravention.
- Any person who seeks the aid of any ultrasound clinic or imaging clinic for sex selection or for conducting prenatal diagnostic techniques on any pregnant women for the purposes other than those specified in Sub-section (2) of Section 4, he shall, be punishable with imprisonment for a term which may extend to 3 years and with fine which may extend to ₹ 50,000 for the first offence and for any subsequent offence with imprisonment which may extend to 5 years and with fine which may extend to ₹ 100,000.

DUTIES OF REGISTERED CENTER

Person conducting ultrasonography on a pregnant woman shall keep complete record thereof in the clinic/center in Form-F and any deficiency or inaccuracy found therein shall amount to contravention of provisions of Section 5 or Section 6 of the Act, unless contrary is proved by the person conducting such ultrasonography.

Facilities or Inspection .... Rule 11

1. Every GCC, GL, Genetic Clinic, Ultrasound Clinic, Imaging Center, Nursing Home, Hospital, Institute or any other place where any of the machines or equipment capable of performing any procedure, technique or prenatal determination of sex or selection of sex before or after conception is used, shall afford all reasonable facilities for inspection of the place, equipment and records to the Appropriate Authority or to any other person authorized by the Appropriate Authority in this behalf for registration of such institutions, by whatever name called, under the Act, or for detection of misuse of such facilities or advertisement, therefore, or for selection of sex before or after conception or for detection/disclosure of sex of fetus or for detection of cases of violation of the provisions of the Act in any other manner.

2. The Appropriate Authority or the officer authorized by it may seal and seize any ultrasound machine, scanner or any other equipment, capable of detecting sex of fetus, used by any organization if the organization has not got itself registered under the Act. These machines of the organizations shall be confiscated and further action shall be taken as per the provision of the Section 23 of the Act. As per Amendment Rule 2011 by Notification dated 31.5.2011.

Intimation of Changes in Employees, Place or Equipment .... Rule 13

Every Genetic Clinic shall intimate every change (addition/removal) of employee, place, address and equipment installed, to the Appropriate Authority within a period of 7 days of such change. As per Delhi High Court order dated 27.6.2012 in CM NO, 8402 of writ petition no. 4009/2012.

New registration not required ....Rule 13

Public Information .... Rule 17

1. Every GCC, GL and Genetic Clinic shall prominently display on its premises a notice in English and in the local language or languages for the information of the public, to effect that disclosure of the sex of the fetus is prohibited under law.

2. At least one copy each of the bare Act and these rules shall be available on the premises of every GCC, GL and Genetic Clinic, and shall be made available to the clientele on demand for perusal.

Code of Conduct .... Rule 18

***Wear NAME TAG yourself and every employee working at the US Clinic. Write full name and designation under signatures**

(Rule 18-VIII and IX)

***Should not indulge in sex determination and female feticide and do not commit any other act of professional misconduct. _____**

(Rule 18-X and XI)

Appeal ....

.. Rule 19

Appeal against charge sheet can be filed to DAC/SAC within 30 days and decision has to be taken within 90 days _____ (Rule 19.1.3)

Maintenance and Preservation of Records ....

.. Rule 9

• Genetic Clinic shall maintain a register showing, in serial order, the names and addresses of the women given genetic counseling, subjected to prenatal diagnostic procedures or prenatal diagnostic tests, the names of their husbands or fathers and the date on which they first reported for such counseling, procedure or test (Rule 9.1)

- For Genetic Counseling Center: Patient records shall be kept as specified in FORM-D (Rule 9.2)
- For Genetic Laboratory: Patient records shall be kept as specified in FORM-E (Rule 9.3)
- For Genetic/US Clinic: Patient records shall be kept as specified in FORM-F (Rule 9.4)
- For Interventional process consent form should be filled FORM-G (Rule 9.5)
- Picture of sonographic image should be preserved in soft/hard copy (Rule 9.6)
- Every Genetic Clinic/Ultrasound Clinic shall send a complete report in respect of all preconception or pregnancy related procedures/techniques/tests conducted by them in respect of each month by 5th day of the following month to the concerned Appropriate Authority even zero report (Rule 9.8).

Search

Whenever an appropriate authority or any other authorized officer has reason to believe that an offence under the Act has been or is being committed, he may search a GCC, a GL or a genetic clinic or any other place which is suspected of conducting prenatal diagnostic techniques.

The scope of the powers of the appropriate authority to search and seize is very wide and it includes the power to:

- Enter freely into the place of search
- Search at all reasonable times
- Examine and inspect all documents like:
  - Registers
  - Records including consent forms, referral slips, charts, laboratory results, microscopic pictures

- Form
- Books
- Pamphlets
- Advertisements
- Material objects like sonographic plates or slides
- Equipment like ultrasonography machines, needles, fetoscope, etc.
- Seize and seal any document, record, material object or equipment, etc. if there is reason to believe that it may furnish evidence of commission of an offence punishable under the Act
- Further, the Appropriate Authority may seal and seize any offending equipment if the facility has not registered itself.

Search and Witnesses

- During the search at least two independent witnesses of the locality should be present
- If no such persons are available or willing to be witness to the search, then two such persons of another locality should be present
- The search should be made in the presence of the two or more independent witnesses
- The witnesses are to be selected by the appropriate authority or the officer duly authorized to conduct search
- The witnesses so selected should be unprejudiced and uninterested as the object of the section is to ensure fair dealing and a feeling of confidence and security amongst public
- The witnesses may be summoned by Court to appear as witnesses
- Any person suspected of having any object with him may also be searched. However, if such person, is a woman than, the search can be done only by a female officer.

Seizure and Preparation of List

- A list of documents, records, material objects, etc. seized during the search should be prepared in duplicate and both copies of such list shall be signed on every page by the appropriate authority or the officer authorized and the witnesses to the seizure

- Assistance of your office staff can always be taken during the process of search and seizure

- The list should be prepared at the place affecting the seizure and if it is not practicable to do so at the place affecting the seizure then for reasons to be recorded in writing it can be done in any other place but it has to be in the presence of the witnesses

- A copy of the list prepared must be handed over to the person from whose custody the document, record or material object, etc. is being seized or his representative under acknowledgment or sent by registered post to him if he is not available at the place of effecting the seizure;

- The person from whose custody the document, record or material object, etc. is being seized or his representative should be permitted to attend during the search and seizure

- The appropriate authority or the officer duly authorized in this behalf may seize any document, material object, record or equipment and take the same into safe custody

- It is preferable that along with the preparation of list of objects seized, a slip is made and pasted on each object seized along with the date, time and the signature of the witnesses

- After a list of seizure is prepared, the same must be sent to the Magistrate having jurisdiction or in charge of the case within 24 hours of the seizure by the appropriate authority or officer duly authorized. Permission to retain the seized objects should be obtained from the Court. The owner of the seized object may make an application to the court for the release of the same. The court may do so after imposing conditions for custody and taking a bond to the effect that, the objects must not be misused for conducting sex-determination tests and that the objects must be produced in Court as and when required, etc.

- Police aid can be taken if the appropriate authority apprehends a law and order problem during the process of search and seizure.

Sealing

- If any material object seized is perishable in nature then arrangements shall be made promptly by the appropriate authority or officer duly authorized for sealing, identification and preservation of the same and send the same to a facility for test if so required
- And till such arrangements for safe removal are made the refrigerator or other equipment used by the GCC, GL or Genetic Clinic for preservation of such material object seized shall be sealed; in case of such sealing it is important to mention the same in the list of seizure prepared;
- If the search and seizure is not completed in a day then the appropriate authority or officer duly authorized may either seal the premises or mount a guard for safe keeping to prevent any tampering of the documents, records, material objects, etc.;
- After seizure the seized objects can be removed to your own premises or may be left in the custody of a respectable person of the locality. If it is not possible to remove the seized objects, they may be retained where they are found after taking a bond from the owner that the same would be produced before the court as and when required.

The appropriate authority is duty bound to maintain systematic records of the search and seizure and the same would also safeguard the appropriate authority against any allegations of abuse.

Collection of Evidence

The evidence that needs to be collected in order to make out a case under the PNDT Act varies depending upon the nature of the violation and in some cases the pieces of evidence can overlap.

Illegal Advertisement

The documentary evidence will include:
- The paper cutting of the advertisement, the name of the newspaper or magazine or any other document which carries the advertisement, the date of the issuance of the advertisement
- The name of the advertiser, his place of business
- The name of the owner of the clinic, center or laboratory issuing such advertisement, the address of the said center, laboratory or clinic
- The name of the distributor, his place of business
- The photograph of the advertisement, the photograph of the hoarding, board, wall on which the advertisement is present, etc.
- The letter heads, memorandum of association, annual reports, statements showing organizational structure and ownership of the newspaper, or 17 Rule 11(2) under the amended PNDT Rules distributorship, or the center. This information has to be collected in order to link the person to the violation.

In Case of Conducting a Test for Determination of Sex or Communication of the Sex of the Fetus

The documentary evidence will include:
- Referral slips
- Consent forms

- Laboratory results
- Microscopic pictures
- Sonographic plates or slides
- Registers containing names and addresses of patients and their families
- Case history of the patient
- Records of clients maintained on the computer or other electronic equipment can be taken on a floppy or a printed copy of the same
- Floppy or printed copy of the ultrasound image of the fetus
- Receipt of fee paid for the test, details of cheque payment, etc.

In Case of Nonregistration, Cancellation or Suspension of Registration

The documentary and oral evidence will include:
- Copy of the registration certificate
- Copy of the affidavit given by the owner that he will not conduct prenatal determination of sex
- Copy of the particulars given about the qualifications of the employees while registration
- Documents collected from the MCI, the degree certificate of the medical practitioners (employees of the center), etc.
- Statements of decoy witnesses
- The tape and video recording
- Other materials collected as evidence in case of conducting tests.

The complete evidence to be submitted before the magistrate would include:
- A copy of the complaint
- A statement showing the list of witnesses both witnesses of the search and seizure and decoy witnesses

- The report of the search and seizure or commonly called Panchnamah
- A copy of the all the documents collected
- Statements of witnesses if any
- Most essential would be the complete address of the GCC, genetic clinic or GL

FORM A

[See Rules 4(1) and 8(1)]
(To be submitted in duplicate)
With supporting documents as enclosures, also in duplicate form of application for registration or renewal of registration of a genetic counseling center/genetic laboratory/genetic clinic

1. Name of the applicant (Specify Shri./Smt./Km./Dr.)
2. Address of the applicant
3. Type of facility to be registered
   (Specify Genetic Counseling Center/Genetic Laboratory/Genetic Clinic/any combination of these)
4. Full name and address/addresses
   (Genetic Counseling Center/Genetic Laboratory/Genetic Clinic with Telephone/Telegraphic Telex/Fax E-mail numbers)
5. Type of ownership and organization
   (Specify individual ownership/partnership/company/cooperative/any other). In case of type of organization other than individual ownership, furnish copy of articles of association and names and addresses of other persons responsible for management, as enclosure.
6. Type of institution
   (Govt. Hospital/Municipal Hospital/Public Hospital/Private Hospital/Private Nursing Home/Private Clinic/Private Laboratory/any other to be stated.)
7. Specific prenatal diagnostic procedures/tests for which approval is sought

(For example amniocentesis, chorionic villi aspiration/chromosomal/biochemical/molecular studies, etc.) Leave blank if registration sought for Genetic Counseling Center only).

8. Equipment available with the make and model of each equipment.

List to be attached on a separate sheet.

9. A. Facilities available in the Counseling Center
   i. Ultrasound
   ii. Amniocentesis
   iii. Chorionic villi aspiration
   iv. Fetoscopy
   v. Fetal biopsy
   vi. Cordocentesis.

   B. Whether facilities are available in the Laboratory/Clinic for the following tests:
   i. Chromosomal studies
   ii. Biochemical studies
   iii. Molecular studies

10. Names, qualifications, experience and registration number of employees may be furnished as an enclosure (Refer Schedules I, II or III).

11. State whether the Genetic Counseling Center/Genetic Laboratory/Genetic Clinic qualifies for registration in terms of minimum requirements laid down in Schedule I, II and III and if not, reasons therefore.

12. For renewal applications only:
    a. Registration No.
    b. Date of issue and date of expiry of existing certificate of registration.

13. List of enclosures:
    Please attach a list of enclosures giving the supporting documents enclosed to this application.
    Date: (.......................................)
    Place, name and signature of applicant

Declaration

1. Sh/Smt/Kum/Dr applicants giving the supporting documents enclosed to this application have read and understood the Prenatal Diagnostic Techniques (Regulation and Prevention of Misuse) Act, 1994 (57 of 1994) and the Prenatal Diagnostic Techniques (Regulation and Prevention of Misuse) Rules, 1995.

2. I also undertake to explain the said Act and Rules to all employees of the Genetic Counseling Center/ Genetic Laboratory/Genetic Clinic in respect of which registration is sought and to ensure that Act and Rules are fully complied with.

   Date: (.......................................)

   Place, name and signature of applicant

Acknowledgement

[See Rules 4(2) and 8(1)]

The application in Form A in duplicate for grant*/ renewal*of registration of Genetic Counseling Center*/Genetic Laboratory*/Genetic Clinic* by_____ (Name and address of applicant) has been received by the Appropriate Authority _____ On (date).

*The list of enclosures attached to the application in Form A has been verified with the enclosures submitted and found to be correct.

OR

On verification, it is found that the following documents mentioned in the list of enclosures are not actually enclosed.

This acknowledgement does not confer any rights on the applicant for grant or renewal of registration.

(.......................................)

Signature and Designation of Appropriate Authority, or authorized person in the Office of the Appropriate Authority.

Date:

Original Seal

Duplicate for Display

FORM B

[See Rules 6(2), 6(5) and 8(2)]

Certificate of Registration

(To be issued in duplicate)

1. In exercise of the powers conferred under Section 19(1) of the Prenatal Diagnostic Techniques (Regulation and Prevention of Misuse) Act, 1994 (57 of 1994), the Appropriate Authority _____ hereby grants registration to the Genetic Counseling Center/Genetic Laboratory* / Genetic Clinic* named below for purposes of carrying out Genetic Counseling/Prenatal Diagnostic Procedures* / Prenatal Diagnostic Tests as defined in the aforesaid Act for a period of five years ending on _____ _

2. This registration is granted subject to the aforesaid Act and Rules thereunder and any contravention thereof shall result in suspension or cancellation of this Certificate of Registration before the expiry of the said period of five years.

   A. Name and address of the Genetic Counseling Centre*/ Genetic Laboratory*/Genetic Clinic*.

   B. Name of Applicant for registration

   C. Prenatal diagnostic procedures approved for (Genetic Clinic).

      i. Ultrasound

      ii. Amniocentesis

      iii. Chorionic villi biopsy

      iv. Fetoscopy

      v. Fetal skin or organ biopsy

    vi. Cordocentesis

    vii. Any other (specify)

D. **Prenatal diagnostic tests* approved (for Genetic Laboratory)**

    i. Chromosomal studies

    ii. Biochemical studies

    iii. Molecular studies

3. Registration No. allotted

4. For renewed certificate of registration only

Period of validity of earlier certificate From .... To .... Or Registration.

Signature, name and designation of The Appropriate Authority

Date:

SEAL

Display one copy of this certificate at a conspicuous place at the place of business.

FORM C

[See Rules 6(3), 6(5) and 8(3)]

Rejection of application for grant/renewal of registration

In exercise of the powers conferred under Section 19(2) of the Prenatal Diagnostic Techniques (Regulation and Prevention of Misuse) Act, 1994, the Appropriate Authority.. hereby rejects the application for grant*/ renewal* of registration of the Genetic Counseling Center*/Genetic Laboratory*/Genetic Clinic* named below for the reasons stated.

Name and address of the Genetic Counseling Center*/Genetic Laboratory*/Genetic Clinic*.................................

Name of Applicant who has applied for registration ....
....

Reasons for rejection of application for registration ....
....

Signature, name and designation
of The Appropriate Authority
Date: Seal
* Strike out whichever is not applicable or necessary.

FORM D

[See rule 9(2)]
Name, Address and Registration No. of Genetic Counseling
Center Record to be Maintained by the Genetic Counseling
Center

1. Patient's name ....
2. Age ....
3. Husband's/Fathers ....
4. Full address with Tel. No., if any ....
5. Referred by (Full name and address of Doctor(s) with
   registration No.(s)) ....
   (Referred note to be preserved carefully with case papers)
   ....
6. Last menstrual period/weeks of pregnancy
7. History of genetic/medical disease in the family (specify)
   basis of diagnosis:
   a. Clinical
   b. Biochemical
   c. Cytogenetic
   d. Other (e.g. radiological)
8. Indication for prenatal diagnosis
   A. Previous child/children with:
      i. Chromosomal disorders
      ii. Metabolic disorders
      iii. Congenital anomaly
      iv. Mental retardation
      v. Hemoglobinopathy
      vi. Sex-linked disorders
      vii. Any other (specify)

    B. Advanced maternal age (35 years)
    C. Mother/father/sibling has genetic disease (specify)
    D. Others (specify)

9. Procedure advised[2]
    i. Ultrasound
    ii. Amniocentesis
    iii. Chorionic villi biopsy
    iv. Fetoscopy
    v. Fetal skin or organ biopsy
    vi. Cordocentesis
    vii. Any other (specify)

10. Laboratory tests to be carried out
    i. Chromosomal studies
    ii. Biochemical studies
    iii. Molecular studies

11. Result of prenatal diagnosis: Normal/abnormal if abnormal, give details.

12. Was MTP advised?

13. Name and address of Genetic Clinic* to which patient referred.

14. Dates of commencement and completion of genetic counseling.

    Date: Name, Signature and Registration No. of the Medical Geneticist/Gynecologist/Pediatrician

FORM E

[See Rule 9(3)]

Name, address and registration no. of genetic laboratory record to be maintained by The genetic laboratory

1. Patient's name
2. Age
3. Husband's/Father's name
4. Full address with Tel. No., if any

5. Referred by/sample sent by (full name and address of Genetic Clinic) (Referral note to be preserved carefully with case papers)

6. Type of sample: Maternal blood/chorionic villus sample/ amniotic fluid/Fetal blood or other fetal tissue (specify)

7. Specify indication for prenatal diagnosis
    A. Previous child/children with
        i.   Chromosomal disorders
        ii   Metabolic disorders
        iii. Malformation(s)
        iv. Mental retardation
        v.   Hereditary hemolytic anemia
        vi. Sex-linked disorder
        vii. Any other (specify)
    B. Advanced maternal age (35 years)
    C. Mother/father/sibling has genetic disease (specify)
    D. Other (specify)

8. Laboratory tests carried out (give details)
    i.   Chromosomal studies
    ii. Biochemical studies
    iii. Molecular studies

9. Result of prenatal diagnosis: Normal/abnormal if abnormal, give details.

10. Date(s) on which tests carried out.

    The results of the prenatal diagnostic tests were conveyed to_____on_____

    Date: Name, Signature and Registration No. of the Medical Geneticist

FORM F

[See Provision to Section 4 (3), Rule 9 (4) and Rule 10 (1A)]
Form for maintenance of records in case of a pregnant woman by genetic clinic/ultrasound clinic/imaging center

Section A: To be filled in for all diagnostic procedures tests

1. Name and complete address of Genetic Clinic/Ultrasound Clinic/Imaging center
2. Registration No. (Under PC and PNDT Act). _____
3. Patient's name_____ Age _____
4. Total Number of living children: Son _____Daughter _____

   a. Number of living sons with age of each living son (in years or months): 1_____2_____ 3_____4_____
   b. Number of living daughters with age of each living daughter (in years or months): 1 ___ 2 ___ 3 ___ 4 ___

5. Husband's/Father's/Mother's Name: _____
6. Full postal address of the patient with contact number, if any:
7. a. Referred by (Full name and address of Doctor(s)/ Genetic Counseling Center): _____ (Referral slips to be preserved carefully with Form F)
   b. Self -referral by Gynecologist/Radiologist/Registered Medical Practitioner conducting the diagnostic procedures
8. Last menstrual period OR weeks of pregnancy: LMP Section B: To be filled in for performing noninvasive diagnostic procedures/tests only
9. Name of the doctor performing the procedure/s: _____ _____
10. Indication/s for diagnostic procedure_____
    a. To diagnose intrauterine and/or ectopic pregnancy and confirm viability.
    b. Estimation of gestational age (dating)
    c. Detection of number of fetus and their chorionicity.
    d. Suspected pregnancy with IUCD in-situ or suspected pregnancy following contraceptive failure/MTP failure.

e. Vaginal bleeding/leaking.
f. Follow-up of cases of abortion.
g. Assessment of cervical canal and diameter of internal os.
h. Discrepancy between uterine size and period of amenorrhea.
i. Any suspected adnexal or uterine pathology/abnormality.
j. Detection of chromosomal abnormalities, fetal structural defects and other abnormalities and their follow-up.
k. To evaluate fetal presentation and position.
l. Assessment of liquor amnii.
m. Preterm labor/preterm premature rupture of membranes.
n. Evaluation of placental position, thickness, grading and abnormalities (placenta previa, retroplacental hemorrhage, abnormal adherence, etc.)
o. Evaluation of umbilical cord-presentation, insertion, nuchal encirclement, number of vessels and presence of true knot.
p. Evaluation of previous cesarean section scars.
q. Evaluation of fetal growth parameters, fetal weight and fetal well-being.
r. Color flow mapping and duplex Doppler studies.
s. Ultrasound guided procedures such as medical termination of pregnancy, external cephalic version, etc. and their follow-up.
t. Adjunct to diagnostic and therapeutic invasive interventions such as chorionic villus sampling (CVS), amniocenteses, fetal blood sampling, fetal skin biopsy, amnio-infusion, intrauterine infusion, placement of shunts, etc.
u. Observation of intrapartum events.
v. Medical/surgical conditions complicating pregnancy.
w. Research/scientific studies in recognized institutions.

11. Procedures carried out (Noninvasive) (Put a "Tick" on the appropriate procedure)
    i. Ultrasound
    ii. Any other (specify)
12. Date on which declaration of pregnant was woman obtained:
13. Date on which procedures carried out: _____
14. Result of noninvasive procedure carried out (report in brief of the test including ultrasound carried out)
    Definite
    Pulse
15. The result of prenatal diagnostic procedures was conveyed to _____ on _____
16. Any indication for MTP as per the abnormality detected in the diagnostic procedures/tests
    Date:
    Place: Doctor Name and Signature
    Section C: To be filled for performing invasive procedures/tests only
17. Name of the doctor/s performing the procedure/s:
    _____
18. History of genetic/medical disease in the family (specify):
    _____
    Basis of diagnosis ("Tick" on appropriate basis of diagnosis):
    a. Clinical
    b. Biochemical
    c. Cytogenetic
    d. Other (e.g. radiological, ultrasonography, etc. specify)
19. Indication/s for the diagnosis procedure ("Tick" on appropriate indication/s):
    A. Previous child/children with:
        i. Chromosomal disorders
        ii. Metabolic disorders

    iii. Congenital anomaly

    iv. Mental Disability

    v. Hemoglobinopathy

    vi. Sex-linked disorders

    vii. Single gene disorder

    viii. Any other (specify)

  B. Advanced maternal age (35 years)

  C. Mother/father/sibling has genetic disease (specify)

  D. Other (specify)

20. Date on which consent of pregnant woman was obtained in Form G prescribed in PC & PNDT Act, 1994:_____

21. Invasive procedures carried out ("Tick" on appropriate indication/s)

    i. Amniocentesis

    ii. Chorionic villi aspiration

    iii. Fetal biopsy

    iv. Cordocentesis

    v. Any other (specify)

22. Any complication/s of invasive procedure (specify)

_____

23. Additional tests recommended (Please mention if applicable)

    i. Chromosomal studies

    ii. Biochemical studies

    iii. Molecular studies

    iv. Preimplantation gender diagnosis

    v. Any other (specify)

24. Result of the procedures/tests carried out (report in brief of the invasive tests/procedures carried out)

_____

25. Date on which procedure carried out:_____

_____

26. The result of prenatal diagnostic procedures was conveyed to _____on _____ _

27. Any indication for MTP as per the abnormality detected in the diagnostic procedures/ tests_____

Date:

Place: Name, Signature and Registration Number with Seal of the Gynecologist/ Radiologist/ Registered Medical Practitioner Performing Diagnostic Procedure/s

Section D: Declaration

Declaration of pregnant woman undergoing ultra-sonography/image scanning

I, Mrs. _____ (name of the pregnant woman) declare that by undergoing ultrasonography/image scanning etc. I do not want to know the sex of my fetus

Date: Signature/Thump impression of pregnant woman

In Case of thumb Impression:

Identified by

(Name) _____ Age: _____ Sex: __ _

Relation (if any): _____ Address and Contact No.: _____ _

Date: Signature of a person attesting thumb impression

Declaration of doctor/person conducting diagnostic procedure/test

I, _____ (name of the person conducting ultrasonography/ image scanning) declare that while conducting ultrasonography/image scanning on Ms. _____ (name of the pregnant woman), I have neither detected nor disclosed the sex of her fetus to anybody in any manner.

Date: Doctor Name, Signature and Seal

FORM G

[See Rule 10]

Form of Consent

I, _____wife/daughter of_____ Age_____years residing at _____hereby state that I have been explained fully the probable side effects and after effects of the prenatal diagnostic procedures. I wish to undergo the prenatal diagnostic procedures in my interest to find out the possibility of any abnormality (i.e. deformity or disorder) in the child I am carrying.

I undertake not to terminate the pregnancy if the prenatal procedure and any prenatal tests conducted show the absence of deformity or disorders. I understand that the sex of the fetus will not be disclosed to me.

I understand that breach of this undertaking will make me liable to penalty as prescribed in the Prenatal Diagnostic Techniques (Regulation and Prevention of Misuse) Act, 1994 (57 of 1994).

Date Signature

Place

I have explained the contents of the above consent to the patient and her companion

(Name _____Address_____) in a language she/they understand.

Name, Signature and Registration number of Gynecologist

Date

Name, Address and Registration number of Genetic Clinic

Relationship

FORM H

[See Rule 9(5)]

Permanent record of application for registration, grant of registration, rejection of application for registration and renewals of registration:

1. Sl. No. _____
_____

2. File number of Appropriate Authority: _____
_____
_____

3. Date of receipt of application for grant of registration:
_____
_____

4. Name, Address, Phone/Fax etc. of Applicant: _____
_____
_____

5. Name and address(es) of Genetic Counseling Center*
   /Genetic Laboratory*/Genetic Clinic*: _____
_____

6. Date on which case considered by Advisory
   Committee and recommendation of Advisory
   Committee, in summary: _____
_____

7. Outcome of application (state granted/rejected and
   date of issue of orders) _____
_____

8. Registration number allotted and date of expiry of
   registration _____

9. Renewals (date of renewal and renewed up to) _____
_____

10. File number in which renewals dealt _____
_____

11. Additional information, if any _____
_____

   Name, Designation and Signature of
   Appropriate Authority
   Guidance for Appropriate Authority
   a. Form H is a permanent record to be maintained
       as a register, in the custody of the Appropriate
       Authority.
   b. *Means strike out whichever is not applicable.

c. Against item 7, record date of issue of order in Form B or Form C.

d. On renewal, the Registration Number of the Genetic Counseling Center/Genetic Laboratory/Genetic Clinic will not change. A fresh registration Number will be allotted in the event of change of ownership or management.

e. No registration number shall be allotted twice.

f. Each Genetic Counseling Center/Genetic Laboratory/ Genetic Clinic may be allotted a folio consisting of two facing pages of the Register for recording Form H.

g. The space provided for 'additional information' may be used for recording suspension, cancellations, rejection of application for renewal, change of ownership/ management, outcome of any legal proceedings, etc.

h. Every folio (i.e. 2 pages) of the Register shall be authenticated by signature of the Appropriate Authority with date, and every subsequent entry shall also be similarly authenticate.

8

CHAPTER

Ergonomics in Reducing Injury Risk in Sonography

DEFINITION

Work-related musculoskeletal disorders (WRMSDs) are defined as injuries that are caused by or aggravated by workplace activities. According to the Department of Labor (DOL), they account for up to 60% of all workplace illnesses, and survey data have shown that approximately 90% of North American sonographers have some form of musculoskeletal disorder (MSD) that can be attributed to their work activities.

Causes and Risk Factors

The causes of MSDs can be attributed to three groups of factors:

- *Biomechanical factors:* Awkward scanning postures, excessive force used in performing an exam, workspace design
- *Faulty work organization:* Infrequent breaks, overtime and on-call incentives, poor employee training
- *Injury management:* Delayed injury reporting and diagnosis, improper injury management, returning worker to injury producing environment

- Work activities that contribute to injuries in sonographers are repetitive motions, forceful exertions or strain, awkward or unnatural positions, uncomfortable positioning of the limbs, static postures, overuse, and frequent reaching above shoulder level.
- There are a number of individual factors that also increase one's risk for an MSD, including sonographer height and weight, age, gender, systemic illnesses, level of physical fitness, and hand dominance.
- Systemic illnesses or injuries that may compromise the blood flow to muscles and tendons increase one's risk for musculoskeletal injury.
- In addition, there are certain leisure activities that can aggravate injury, such as playing musical instruments, running, sewing and racket sports. These activities put extra strain on the muscles of the hands and forearm and the intervertebral discs of the back.
- The use of filmless storage in sonography has contributed to the increase in MSDs because this now allows sonographers to move rapidly from patient to patient without sufficient rest periods.
- The use of narrow transducers for certain examinations requires a tighter "pinch" grip that causes excess stress on the fingers and forearm muscles.
- Chairs or stools and examination tables that are not adjustable result in sonographers using excessive reach and trunk twist to access the patient during an examination.
- Increases in workloads are due to downsizing, shortages of skilled sonographers, and increased demand for exams. Thus, each sonographer is performing more patient examinations during the workday, often necessitating more overtime and fewer work breaks, thus resulting in less recovery time.

Symptoms

Symptoms of musculoskeletal injury are as follows:

- Pain
- Inflammation
- Swelling
- Loss of sensation
- Numbness
- Tingling
- Burning
- Clumsiness
- Muscle spasm.

Symptoms of an MSD can occur after months or years of overuse and have been staged according to their reversibility and outcome.

Stage 1: Aching and fatigue that subside with overnight rest and do not result in a reduction in work performance

Stage 2: Recurrent aching and fatigue that do not subside with overnight rest; symptoms occur earlier in the workday and affect performance at work.

Stage 3: Aching, fatigue, and weakness result in reduced performance in work and leisure activities; pain occurs with nonrepetitive movements; symptoms disturb sleep and may last years.

Types of Musculoskeletal Disorders

Specific disorders of MSDs are as follows:

- *Tenosynovitis/tendonitis*: Inflammation of the tendon sheath and tendon
- *Carpal tunnel syndrome*: Entrapment of the median nerve due to inflammation and edema of the soft tissues in the carpal tunnel of the wrist
- *Cubital tunnel syndrome*: Entrapment of the ulnar nerve due to inflammation of the soft tissues in the elbow

- *Thoracic outlet syndrome*: Compression of the subclavian vessels and brachial plexus against the scalene muscle or the first rib
- *Trigger finger*: Inflammation of the tendon sheath of a finger, entrapping the tendon within and preventing flexion and/or extension of the finger
- *de Quervain disease*: Tendonitis specific to the thumb
- *Lateral/medial epicondylitis*: Inflammation of the epicondyles of the distal humerus caused by repeated twisting of the forearm and exerting pressure with the arm.
- Rotator cuff injury
- Bursitis of the shoulder
- *Thoracic outlet syndrome:* Entrapment of the brachial plexus and/or the subclavian vessels by the muscles of the chest or the first rib
- *Spinal degeneration:* Caused by constrained postures causing increased pressure between the vertebrae of the spine
- *Neck/back sprains:* Caused by standing or sitting in awkward postures during an examination.

Muscle Physiology

- Muscles and tendons are designed to be used regularly, but when frequency and duration of loading exceed the ability of the muscles and tendons to adapt, inflammation occurs followed by degeneration, microtears, and scar formation.
- This type of stress is a function of the transducer time a sonographer maintains daily, particularly when repeatedly performing the same type of examination.
- Work pace, recovery time, and level of muscular effort lead to these injuries.
- Muscles require an adequate supply of oxygen to function properly. Oxygen is pumped into muscles, and wastes are removed through the normal contraction of muscles during dynamic movement.

- Static postures prevent this process from occurring, resulting in decreased oxygen to the muscles and a buildup of lactic acid followed by fatigue and potential injury.
- Nerve damage results from arm abduction, flexion, and extension of the wrist and/or fingers. These motions cause swelling of the soft tissues that compress and entrap the nerves of the wrist or fingers.

Impact of Musculoskeletal Disorders

The impact of MSDs ranges from minor discomfort to career-ending injury. There are a number of emotional and financial implications for the injured worker as well as an impact on the employer, coworkers, and workers' compensation.

Treatment

Once an accurate diagnosis of musculoskeletal injury has been made, treatment ranges from analgesics and anti-inflammatory medications to surgery. However, treatment of work-related MSDs has a poor outcome because sonographers are often expected to return to the same work environment that caused the injury initially. It is important, therefore, to *prevent* injury by addressing the risk factors in the workplace

Injury Prevention

- The keys to prevention are *education and ergonomics.*
- Exam gloves with textured fingers, which make it easier to grip the transducer, should be available in various sizes.
- Equipment manufacturers continue to develop ergonomic transducer shapes, lighter cables, and adjustable control panels and monitors. These features should be considered when purchasing new ultrasound systems.
- Scanning rooms can be ergonomically designed to fit each individual sonographer with attention to room layout and

proper lighting. Engineering controls, which address the physical hazards present in the workplace, are the most effective means for reducing and, in some instances, eliminating WRMSDs.

Individual Prevention Methods

- Sonographers must learn to change the behaviors that have led to pain in the past. This can be done by using adjustable chairs or stools with backs and height-adjustable examination tables.

- Taking the time to position the equipment and the patient close to them can significantly reduce reaching and twisting. Attention should be given to arranging a patient's room during bedside examinations so that the sonographer can scan the patient comfortably without excessive reach or abduction of his or her upper extremities.

- The simple practice of taking multiple "mini breaks," stopping to relax the neck and shoulder muscles, opening and closing hands, and resting the eyes can make a significant difference in the level of muscle strain and fatigue.

- Using arm support devices, such as cushions, to support the scanning arm drastically reduces the amount of muscle activity—in the arm, thus reducing fatigue and risk for injury.

- Sonographers should also learn to perform stretching and strengthening exercises designed to condition the shoulder, arms, and hands.

- During an acute injury, it is recommended that any leisure activities that aggravate the pain be limited.

Departmental Changes

- Department managers should encourage sonographers to take rest breaks during the workday.

- Examinations should be scheduled so that the same examinations are not scheduled together, thus reducing repetitive motions.
- Employees should be instructed in the proper use of all examination room equipment.
- Bedside examinations should be reserved for those patients whose condition makes it impossible for them to leave the nursing floor. Bedside exams should be scheduled so that they are shared among staff members rather than assigned to one person all day.
- Ideally, a hospital transporter should be used for the transport of hospital patients to the ultrasound department.
- However, if the policy of a facility is to perform all inpatient exams portable, it is recommended that a room be provided on the floor that is specifically equipped for ultrasound exams. This can be a small room without windows that has an electrically adjustable exam table and suitable chair as well as an ultrasound system with ergonomic features or an adjustable stand or cart on which a hand-carried ultrasound system can be placed.

Ergonomic Principles

Ergonomics is the science of designing a job to best fit the body of an individual worker, which ultimately leads to improved operator productivity. Current equipment designs, from ultrasound equipment to examination room tables and chairs, incorporate more ergonomic principles, designed with the sonographers safety as a priority.

Ergonomic Equipment

- The ultrasound system should have a height-adjustable monitor that swivels and tilts.

- The control panel should also be height-adjustable and move independent of the monitor. Frequently used keys should be positioned so that minimal reach is needed to access them. Transducers should be easy to exchange and connect. The system should be easy to move position and should have brakes.

- The examination table should also be electrically height-adjustable and easy to move. The height range should be between 22 and 40 in. The table width should be between 24 and 27 in, although a wider table may be necessary for larger patient populations. If there are side rails on the table, they should retract completely below and beneath the table so that there is no additional distance between the sonographer and the patient.

- An ergonomic examination room chair, rich is often overlooked when designing ultrasound facilities, is extremely important in contributing to injury prevention. The chair should have an adjustable seat pan, allowing sonographers of different heights to have good support for their thighs. It should be height-adjustable and capable of rising high enough to allow for a sit-stand position. It should have five or more casters for stability, a foot rest, and lumbar support. The back of the chair should also be adjustable to accommodate workers of different heights. A saddle-shaped design for the seat of the chair has been shown to promote the most upright and comfortable posture.

- Sonographers should use arm support during an examination to prevent the upper extremity muscles from supporting the entire weight and activity of the arm. This support can range from rolled-up towels to cushions to more sophisticated arm support devices. Although initially an economic solution, rolled-up towels incur a significant laundry expense.

Ergonomic Adaptations of Current Equipment

- Newer equipment designs incorporate ergonomic principles that may not be available in existing examination room equipment.
- Injury prevention is most effectively achieved by the purchase and use of ergonomically designed chairs, examination tables, and ultrasound systems.
- There are a number of ways that it can be made more ergonomic or used in a more ergonomically correct way. Injuries can be minimized in a number of ways.
- For examination room chairs with heights that cannot be adjusted, something can be added to the chair, such as a folded towel, a lumbar support cushion, or an air-filled seat cushion.
- Standing up while scanning may allow the sonographer to maintain a more comfortable posture and places less compression force on the spine than does sitting in a poorly designed chair. The key is for sonographers to position themselves high enough to reduce the reach and abduction of the scanning arm.
- Working with current examination tables requires that the patient be positioned close to the sonographer. This prevents unnecessary reaching and arm fatigue.
- While it may be helpful to sit on the bed with the patient, especially in those cases when the patient cannot move to the edge, great care must be taken to check that there are no needles or other sharp objects accidently left in the sheets.
- An electrically height-adjustable table is critical in reducing the risk for injury to the upper extremity and neck. Fixed-height tables do not allow the sonographer to make the adjustments necessary to reduce the abduction of his or her scanning arm. For examination tables that are not height-adjustable, mattresses can be added or subtracted in an attempt to obtain an optimal height.

- Neck and upper extremity structures can be scanned with the patient seated in a wheelchair or a chair with arms, thus allowing the sonographer to get closer to the patient and maintain a more comfortable position.
- If the monitor on the ultrasound system is stationary, the engineering department of the hospital or ultrasound facility may be able to modify the monitor of the ultrasound equipment to make it height- adjustable.
- This significantly lengthens the time needed to complete the study and would work against productivity.
- For equipment with fixed height monitors; a small, auxiliary monitor may be added on top of the equipment for viewing examinations while standing.

Changes in Scanning and Workstation Practices

Bedside Examinations

Try to share these examinations with other colleagues in the department and do portable examinations only when absolutely necessary, not because it is just more convenient.

Computer Equipment

- Most departments use picture-archiving and communication system (PACS) for image storage and separate computers for generating reports.
- Placement of this equipment can be as important as the equipment *in* the examination rooms.
- Place the PACS 2nd computer towers so that there is free leg room under the table.
- Try to obtain a height adjustable chair or make the adjustments to the chair to keep arms in a neutral position to the body.
- Ideally, the computer monitors should be mounted on articulated arms so that their positions can be changed if necessary.

- However, an easy solution is to place the monitor on something to raise it to eye level. Note the position of the key-board, and raise it to a comfortable position, keeping it close. The mouse should also be positioned close to eliminate reaching.
- It is important that sonographers take responsibility for how they practice the profession.

Breaks

Take lunch breaks. Do not give this up to accommodate add-on patients just to leave work on time at the end of the day; the muscle recovery time achieved by taking a break is more important.

Scanning Practices

- Use mild transducer pressure.
- Do not be "image-driven." Avoid sacrificing musculoskeletal health for a textbook picture that does not impact the diagnosis.
- Use a light grip on the transducer and use textured-finger gloves that fit properly when possible. This improves the grip on the transducer, thus reducing the force required to hold it.
- If the transducer is so narrow that it requires a pinch grip to hold it, try to use adaptive products that can be slipped over the transducer to widen it. Or try a different way of holding the transducer that lessens the need to pinch it.
- Support your scanning arm by placing support cushions or a rolled-up towel under the elbow or by using an arm support device.
- When performing transvaginal examinations, position the equipment at the foot end of the examination table and sit or stand between the patient's legs with your scanning arm supported on towels or a cushion resting on your thigh.

- Cardiac exams should be performed from the patient's left side.
- When performing lower extremity vascular exams, those patients who are compliant should be instructed on how to dorsiflex the foot to perform self-augmentation of blood flow, thus reducing the need for the sonographers to twist and reach across their bodies in order to manually perform augmentation.
- The patient should be repositioned after the right leg has been scanned so that the left leg is now closer to the sonographer .
- Another option is to raise the table to its maximum height and have the patient dangle his or her legs over the side toward you. Place a towel on your thigh and then place the patient's foot on the towel. You can now manually perform compression-causing augmentation without abducting or crossing your arms.
- When performing carotid exams, you can reduce reach and arm abduction by scanning from the head of the exam table. Another option is scan the patient while he or she is seated.

SELF-CARE

- Practice strengthening exercises regularly at home to strengthen arm and shoulder muscles.
- Stretch before starting to scan each day.
- Exercise putty or a large rubber band can be used for hand-stretching exercises to increase blood supply to the hand and fingers.
- Take mini breaks during patient examinations. Mini breaks require only a few seconds and add only approximately two minutes to each examination.
- Put the transducer down and relax your scanning arm and hand. Gently shake the hand and arm, open and close your fist, and close your eyes momentarily.

- Get plenty of rest and practice good nutrition.
- Have your eyes examined to ensure that corrective lenses are appropriately adjusted for an 18- to 22-in screen distance. This helps reduce eyestrain and headaches and prevents the need to lean closer to the monitor.
- Room lighting should be easy to reach from the scanning location and should have dimming capabilities. Make sure the examination room lighting is adjusted to prevent glare on the monitor.
- When you have an acute injury, try to limit the time spent on a home computer, and especially avoid a lot of mouse work or graphics all at one time.
- Limit leisure activities that use the upper extremity, such as gardening, needlework, knitting, playing musical instruments, and racket sports.
- It is imperative that you become aware of your work postures and make changes as soon as you notice strain and fatigue.

3D in Obstetric Imaging (The World is Changing)

Contributed by Prof Ritsuko K Pooh & Prof Asim Kurjak
(Images reproduced with permission)

THE INTERNET REVOLUTION

The number of web pages doubling exponentially 3 times a year (a factor of 8).
Every day:

- 3 million new web pages
- 10 billion instant messages
- 19 billion e-mail messages

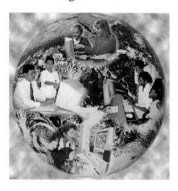

- 12 billion spam messages
- 80% web sites that will exist in a year (from now)—do not exist.

Adaptation is Essential for Survival

"It is not the strongest of the species that survive, nor the most intelligent, but the one most responsive to change".
–Charles Darwin

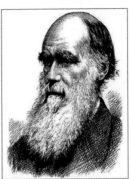

The Dilemma is Rather Old

Socrates himself feared that writing, the oldest information-technology of all, might end up making us less intelligent, with reading substituting for remembering.

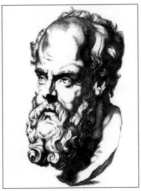

Source: http://www.dailymail.co.uk/sciencetech/article-1284564/

We Need to Think "Scientifically"

To survive in the modern age, you need to think 'scientifically' (even if you are not a scientist), to be able to put things into categories, to operate machines, to think in a linear fashion and use modern technology.

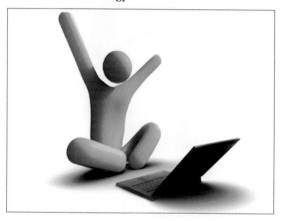

Source: http://www.dailymail.co.uk/sciencetech/article-1284564/

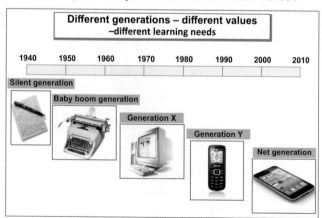

The Beliefs of Great Philosopher Socrates

"The secret of change is to focus all of your energy, not on fighting the old, but on building the new."   *–Socrates*

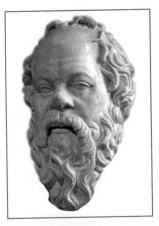

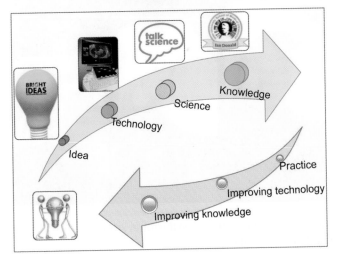

Imaging

Our culture is growing more global. While it still relies on words, they are increasingly wrapped up with images, and it is images people remember.

3D Ultrasound

20 years of development.

HDlive Silhouette

Changes of the Acoustic Impedance within the Volume

Organ boundaries, vessel walls, fluid filled cavities, have a big and abrupt change of the acoustic impedance. At those changes within the tissue, at those "edges" so to say, the Silhouette algorithm creates a gradient.

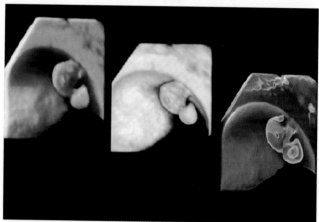

Source: http://www.fetal–medicine-pooh.jp

Look through the volume, see the inner structures just like with a body made of glass.

An image of **a twin pregnancy at 8.5 weeks** given by the Voluson E10 ultrasound.

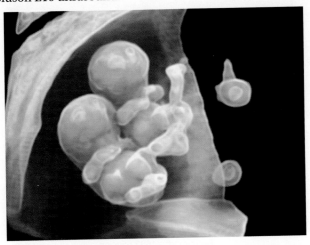

An image of **a DC DA twin pregnancy at 8.5 weeks** given by the Voluson E10 ultrasound HDlive Silhouette

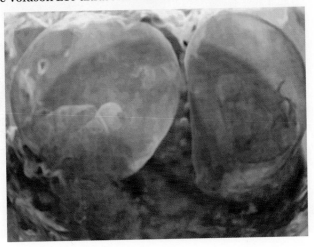

One Picture is Worth a Thousand Words

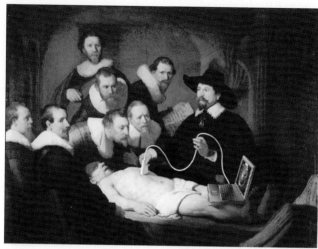

Rembrandt's 1632 painting
"The Antomy Lesson of Dr. Nicolaes Tulp"

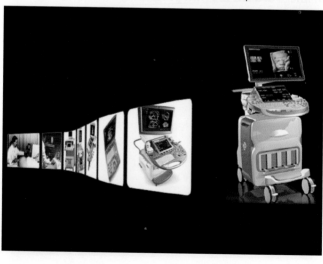

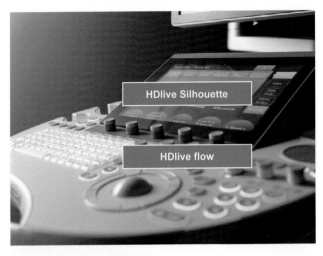

HDlive Silhouette HDlive Flow in the Early Pregnancy (6–10 Weeks of Gestation)

6 Weeks

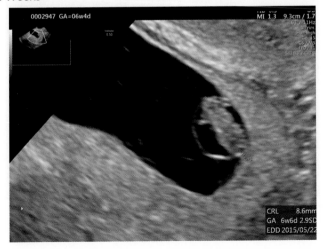

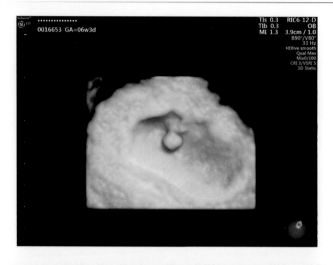

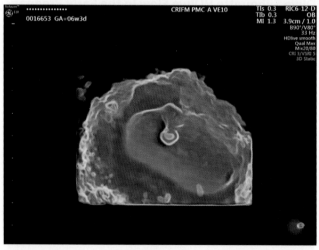

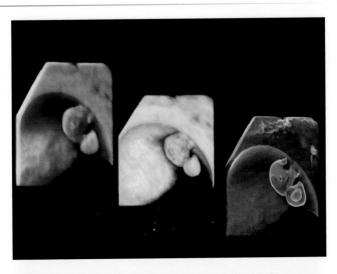

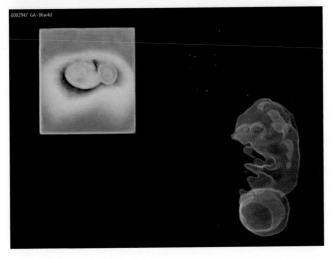

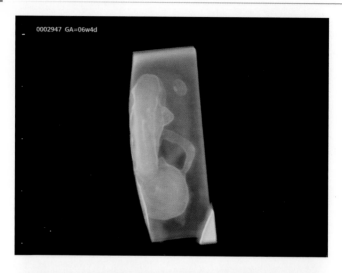

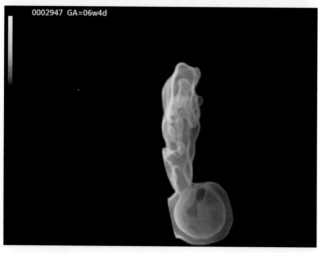

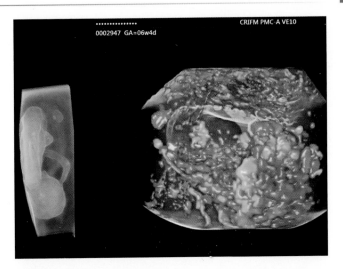

7 Weeks

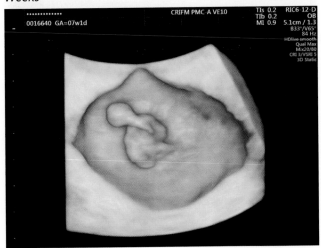

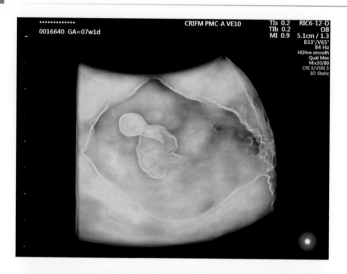

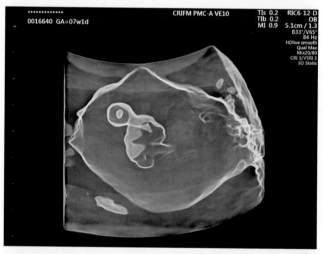

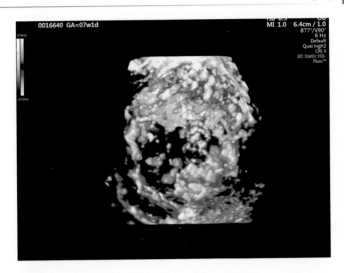

8 Weeks

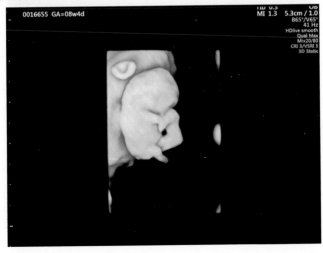

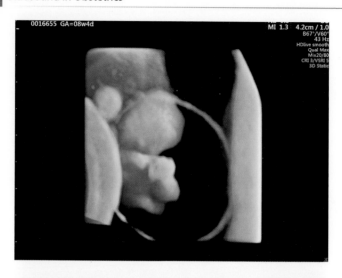

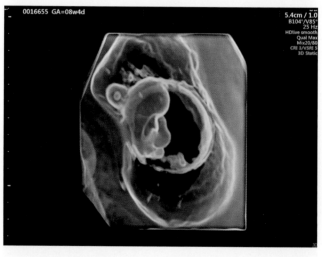

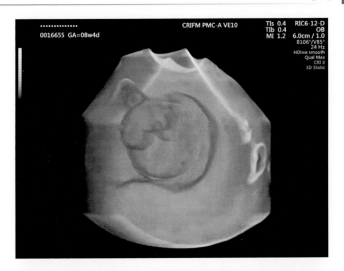

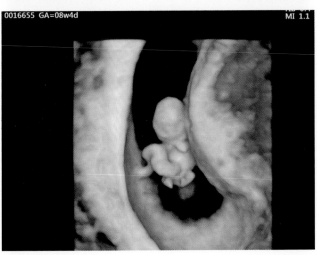

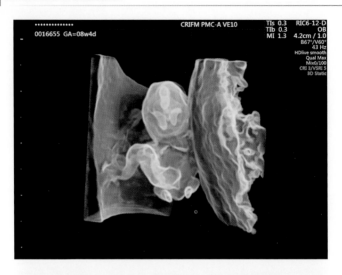

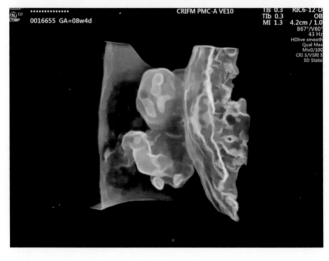

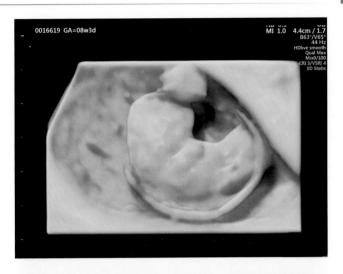

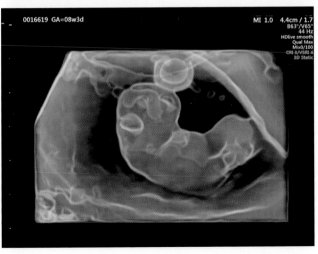

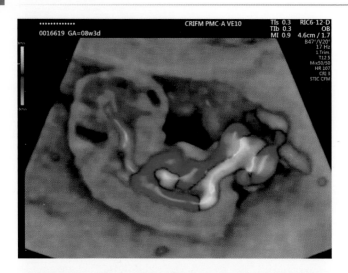

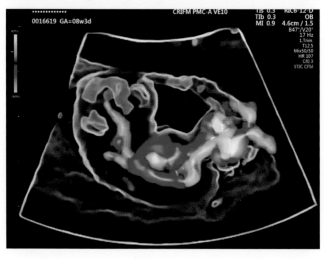

9 Weeks

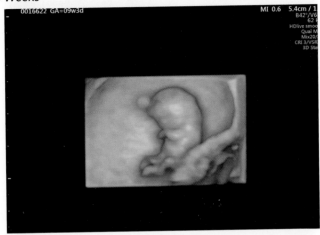

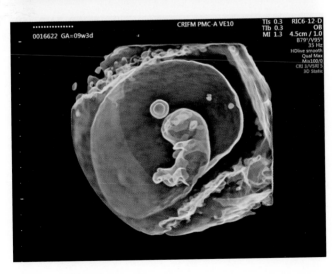

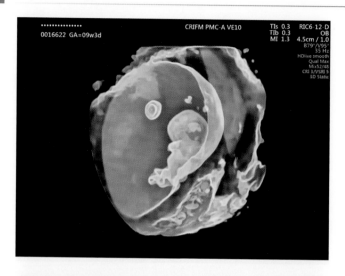

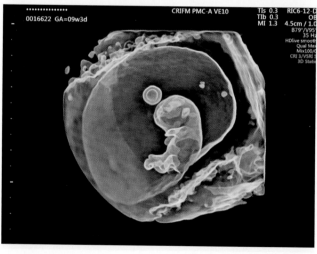

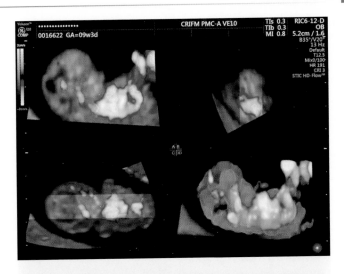

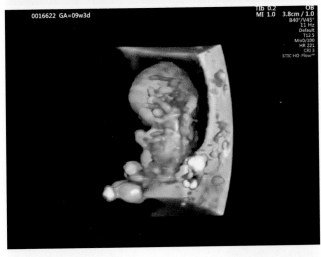

10 Weeks

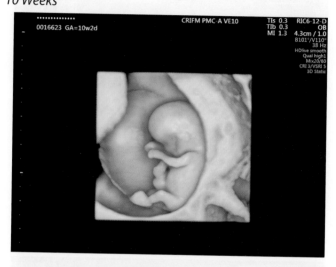

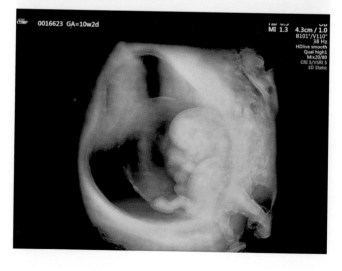

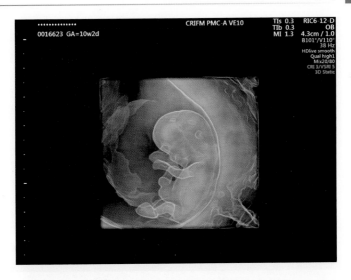

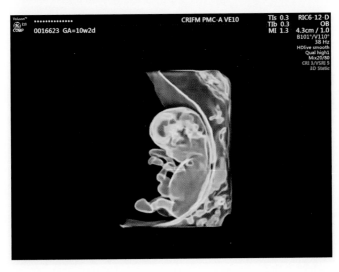

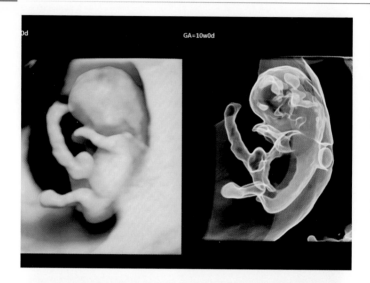

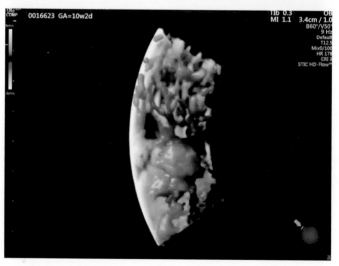

HDlive Silhouette HDlive Flow in the 1st Trimester (11–13 Weeks of Gestation)

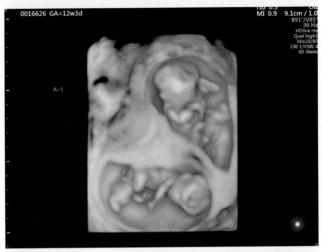

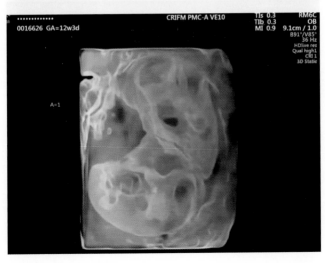

Prune Belly Syndrome

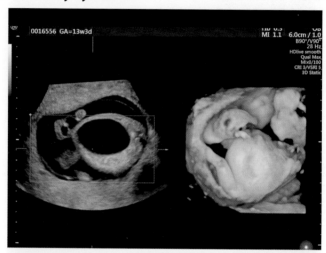

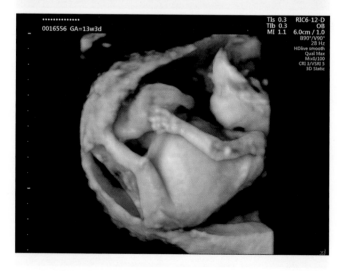

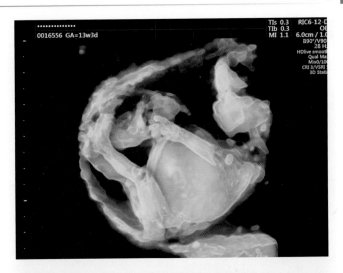

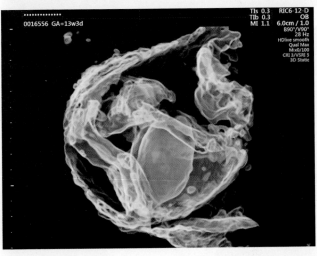

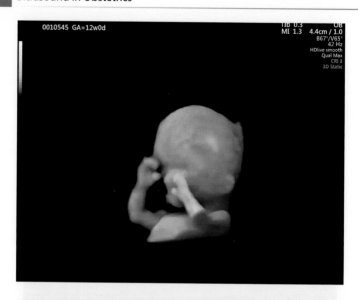

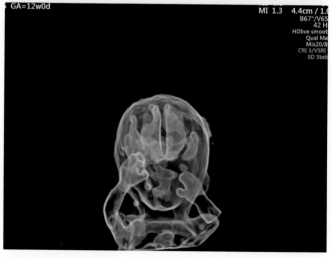

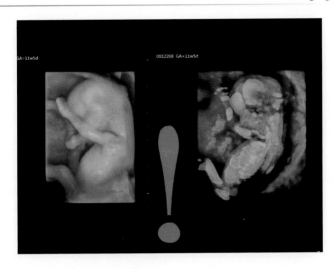

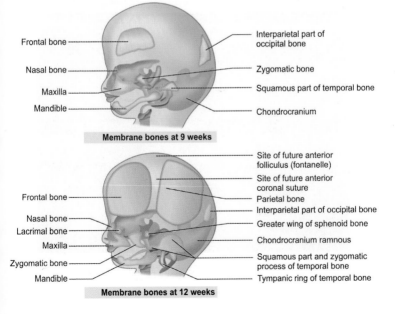

Frontal bone

Nasal bone

Maxilla

Mandible

Interparietal part of occipital bone

Zygomatic bone

Squamous part of temporal bone

Chondrocranium

Membrane bones at 9 weeks

Site of future anterior folliculus (fontanelle)

Site of future anterior coronal suture

Parietal bone

Interparietal part of occipital bone

Greater wing of sphenoid bone

Chondrocranium ramnous

Squamous part and zygomatic process of temporal bone

Tympanic ring of temporal bone

Frontal bone

Nasal bone

Lacrimal bone

Maxilla

Zygomatic bone

Mandible

Membrane bones at 12 weeks

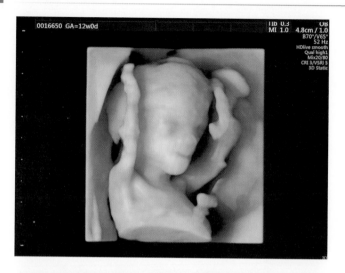

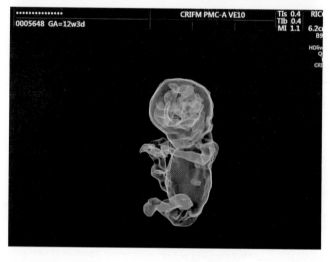

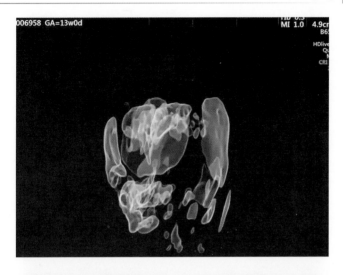

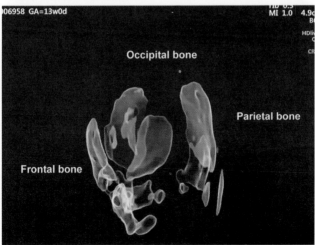

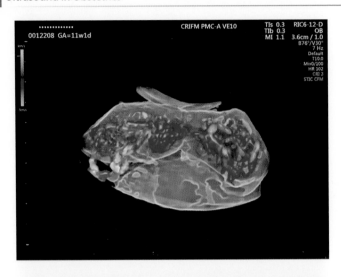

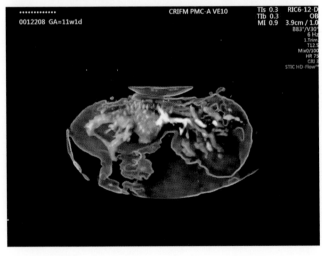

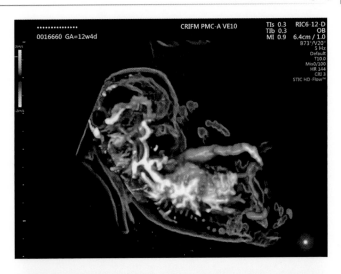

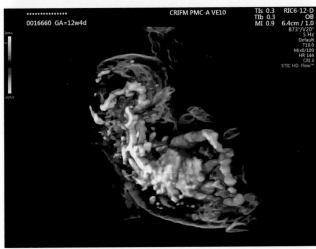

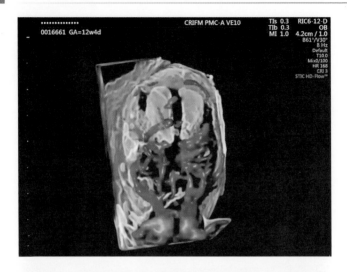

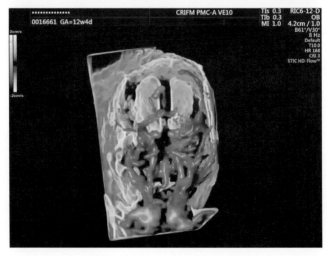

Pulmonary Artery and Vein

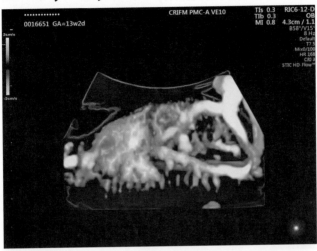

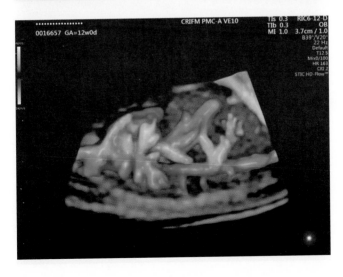

13 Weeks Brain Vascularity

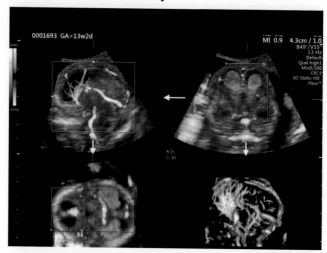

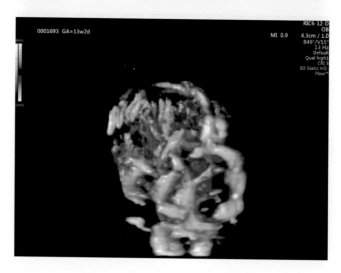

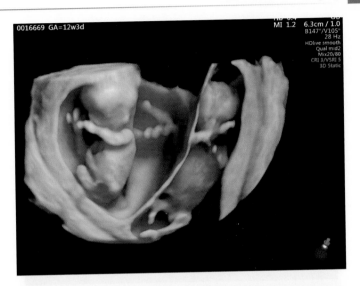

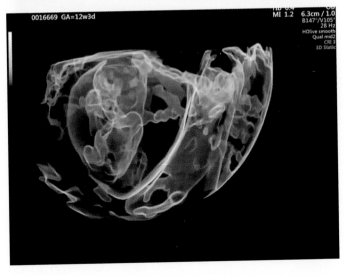

12 Weeks Velamentous Cord Insertion

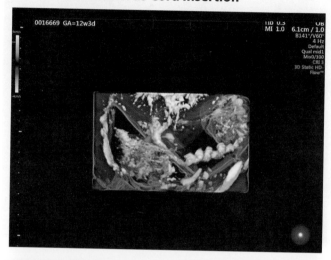

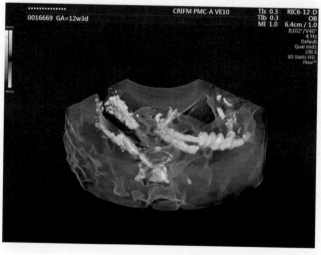

12 Weeks Normal Heart

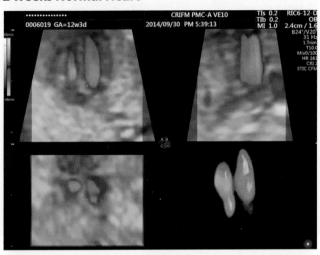

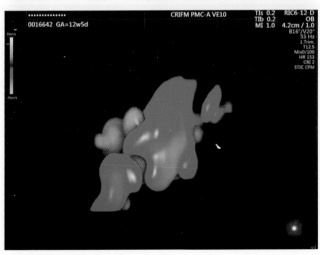

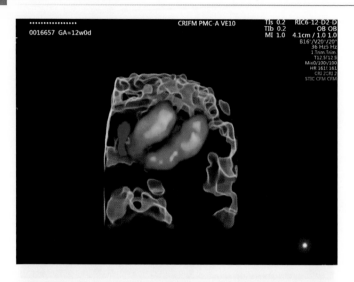

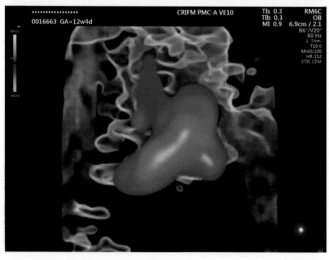

13 Weeks Normal Heart

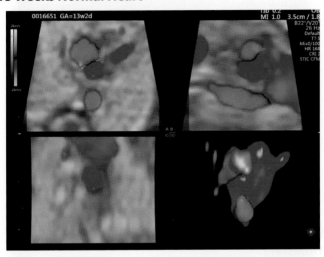

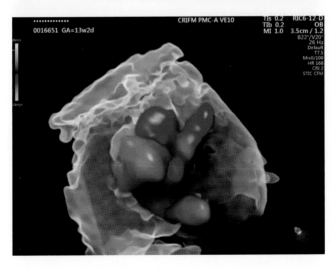

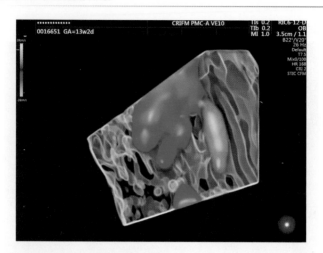

HDlive Silhouette HDlive Flow in the 2nd and 3rd Trimesters

Detection of Cystic Area

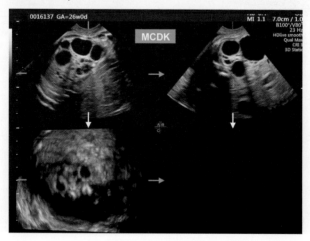

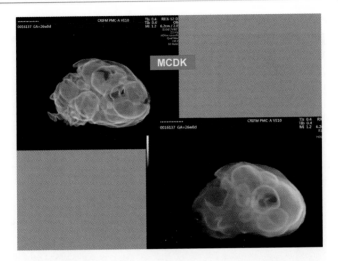

Vascularity to MCDK

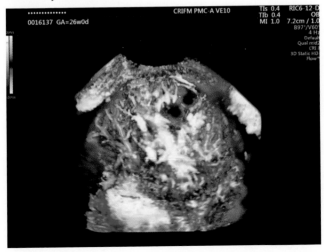

16 Weeks, DWM and Ventriculomegaly

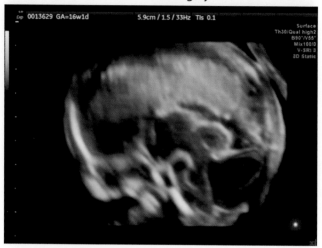

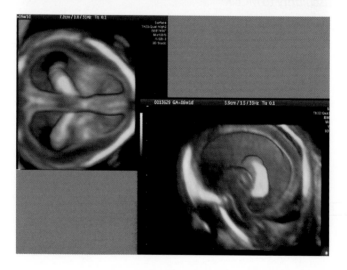

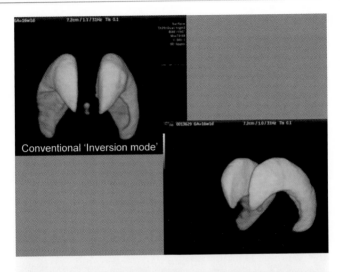

Conventional 'Inversion mode'

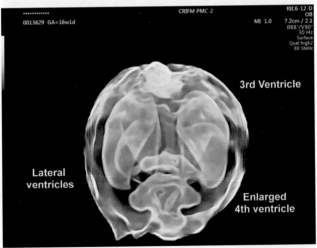

14 Weeks Holoprosencephaly, Semilobar Type

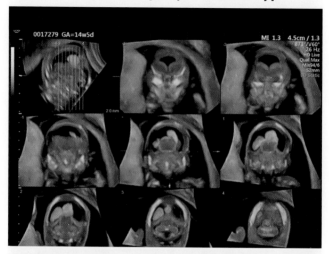

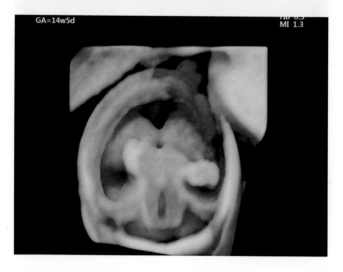

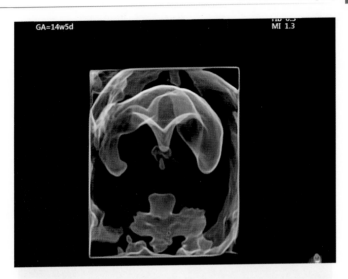

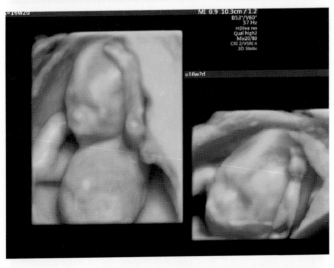

16 Weeks Anterior Fontanelle

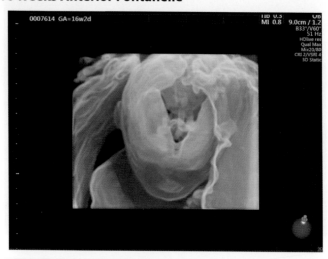

20 Weeks Vertebrae and Ribs

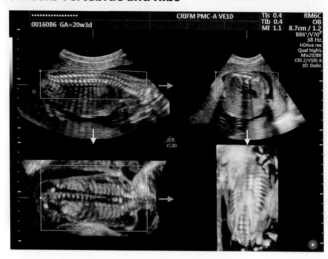

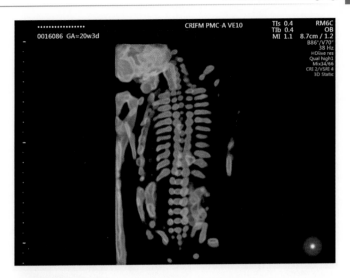

20 Weeks Cervical Vertebrae

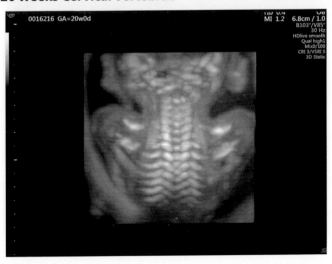

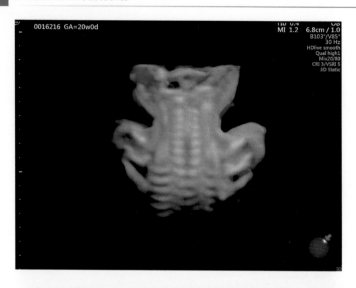

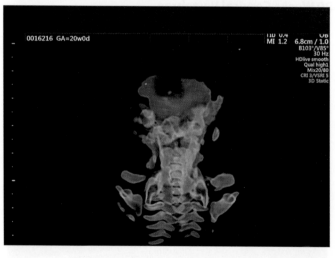

18 Weeks Vertebrae and Ribs

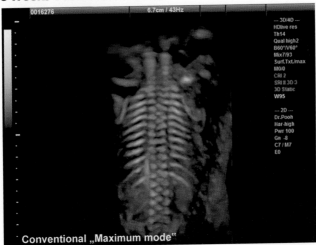

Conventional „Maximum mode"

18 Weeks Vertebrae (P-A View)

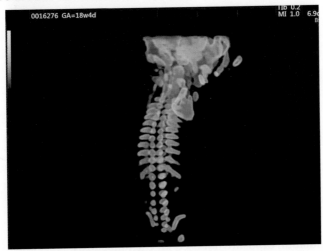

18 Weeks Vertebrae (P-A View)

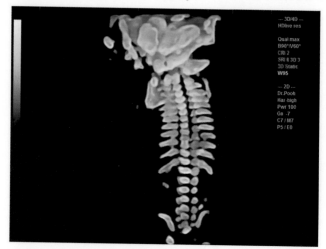

Fetal 3D-CT for Skeletal Dysplasia

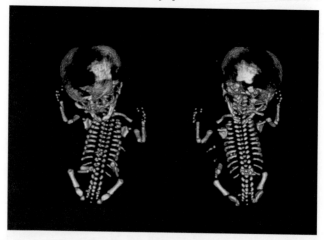

Radiation exposure not used for early diagnosis.

18 Weeks Vertebrae (A-P view)

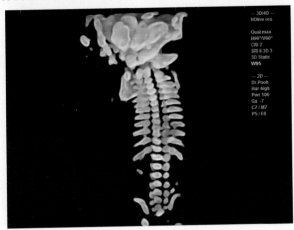

Noninvasive technology useful for early diagnosis

HDlive Silhouette

Investigation of Skeletal System Diseases

Umbilical cord Insertion

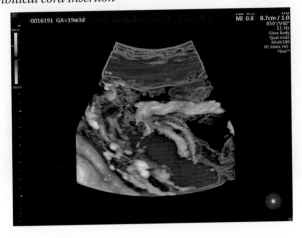

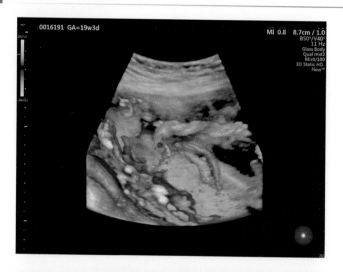

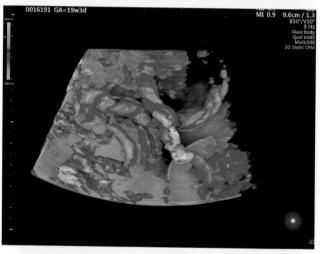

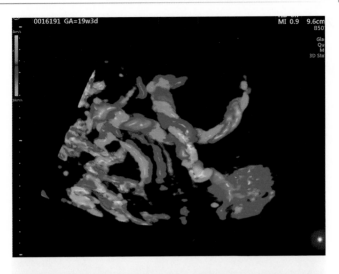

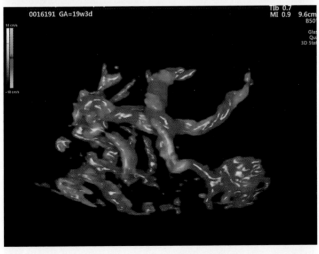

21 Weeks Umbilical Artery Aneurysm

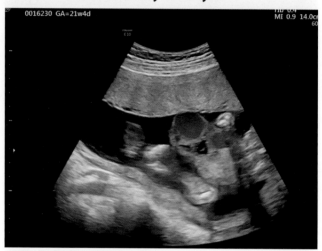

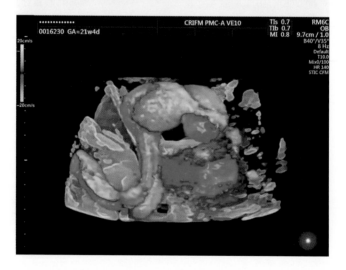

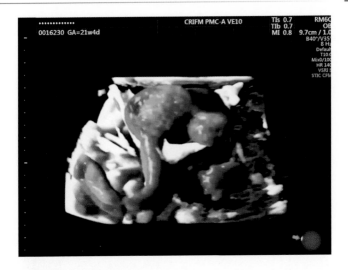

18 Weeks Normal Heart

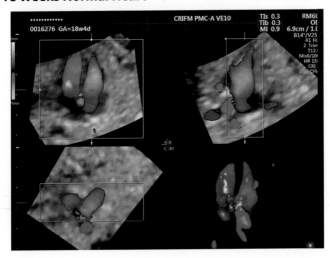

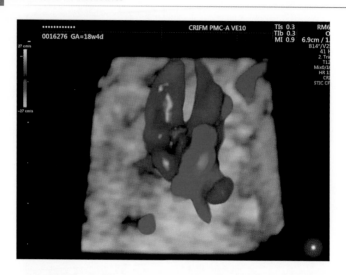

20 Weeks Pulmonary Artery and Vein

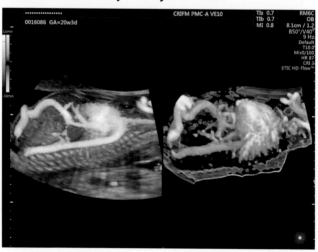

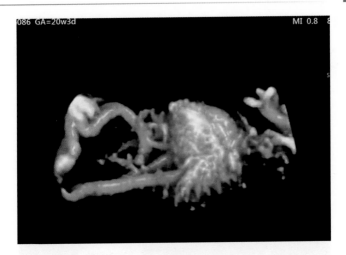

Hyaloid Artery (*see in fetuses and premature babies*)

97% of mature infants: No remnant HA is visible

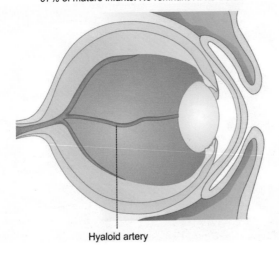

Hyaloid artery

19 Weeks Eyeball

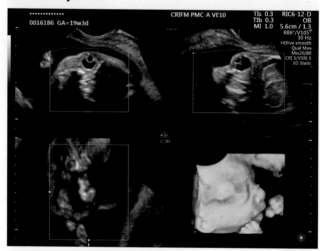

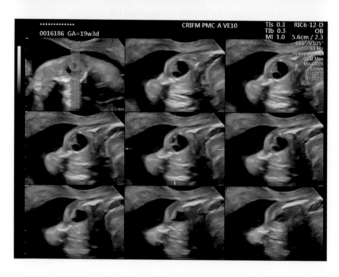

19 Weeks Eyeball and Lens

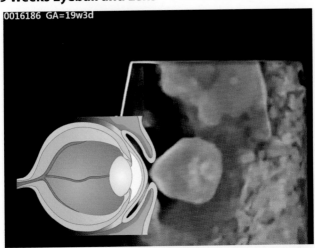

19 Weeks Eye Vascularity

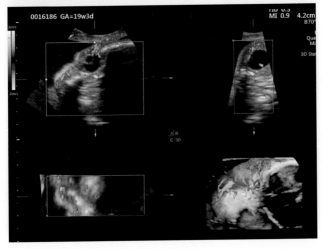

19 Weeks Hyaloid Artery

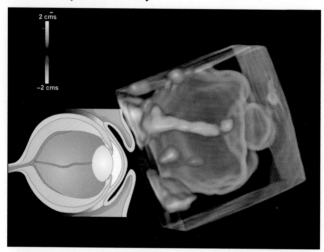

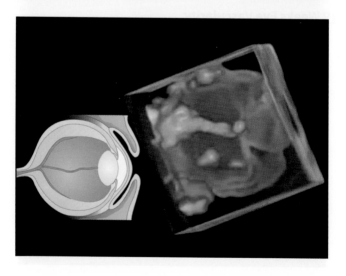

16 Weeks Eyeball

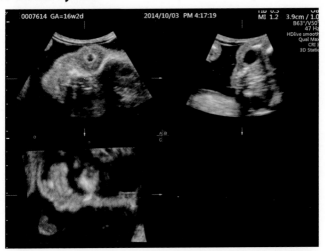

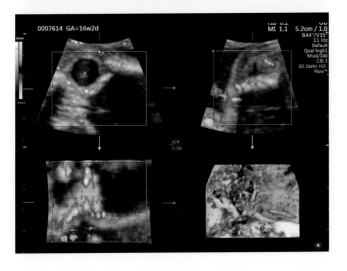

16 Weeks Hyaloid Artery

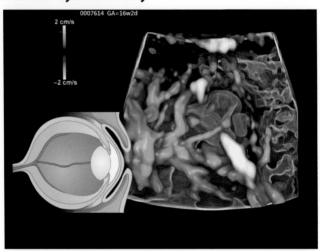

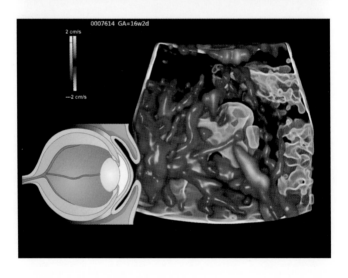

20 Weeks Brain Vascularity

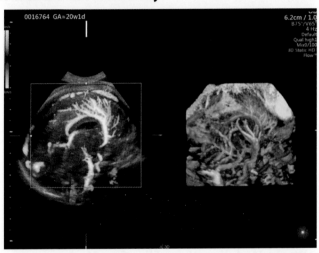

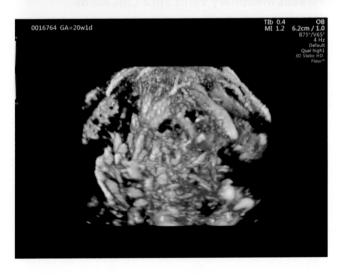

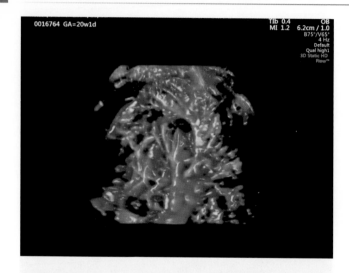

29 Weeks Medullary Veins Slice Cine Mode

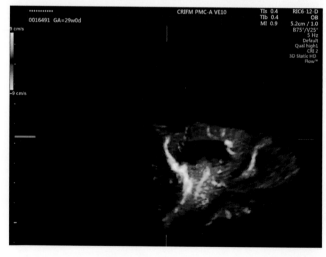

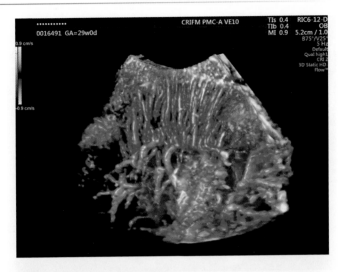

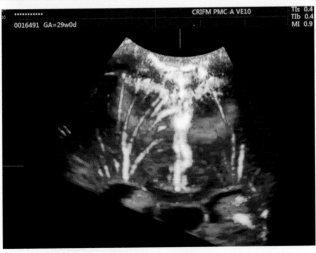

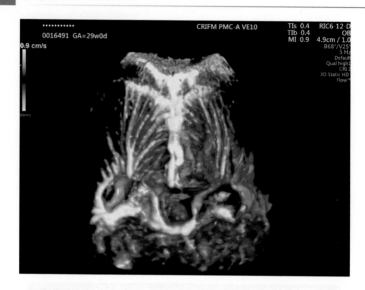

More Clinical Information than Molecular Genetical Technology

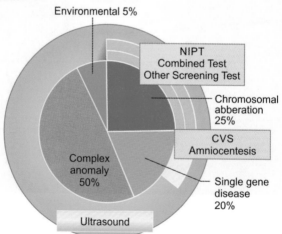

Noninvasive Direct-viewing All-inclusive Technology

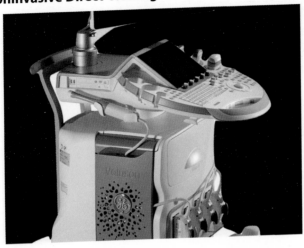

First Modality of Prenatal Diagnosis with Infinite Potential

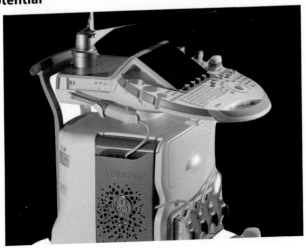

Fetus First should be our Priority

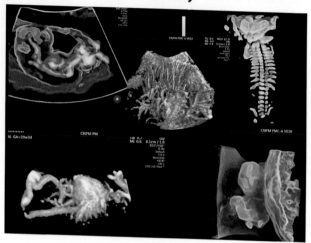

The authors of step by step series are extremely grateful to Prof Ritsuko K Pooh and Prof Asim Kurjak, Directors of Ian Donald school for contributed this chapter.

Appendices

Normal Values

NUCHAL TRANSLUCENCY

- Nuchal translucency thickness usually increases with gestational age.
- 1.5 mm and 2.5 mm are the 50th and 95th percentile respectively for gestational ages between 10 and 12 weeks.
- 2.0 mm and 3.0 mm are the 50th and 95th percentile respectively for gestational ages between 12 and 14 weeks.

NUCHAL SKIN FOLD

- 14–18 weeks: Normal value <04 mm, borderline 04–05 mm and >05 mm requires further karyotypic analysis
- 18–22 weeks: Normal value <05 mm, borderline 05–06 mm and > 06 mm requires further karyotypic analysis.
- After 22 weeks the sensitivity of nuchal skin fold thickness measurement for predicting karyotypic abnormalities is poor.

RENAL PELVIS

- The values for the anteroposterior diameter of the renal pelvis (measured on a transverse view through the kidney)
- From 15–20 weeks of gestation < 04 mm is normal, 04-07 mm is borderline and > 08 mm is abnormal or hydronephrotic.
- From 20 weeks onwards <06 mm is normal, 06–09 is borderline and >10 mm is abnormal or hydronephrotic.
- Borderline cases are to be reviewed by serial scans before labelling them as hydronephrotic. Check for caliectasis or ureteric dilatation.

VENTRICULAR ATRIUM

- The width of the body, anterior horn and posterior horn of the lateral ventricle are taken.
- Normal value <08 mm, borderline 08–10 mm and >10 mm abnormal.

CEREBELLAR TRANSVERSE DIAMETER

The CTD in mm from 14–22 weeks is equal to the gestational age of the fetus in weeks.

CISTERNA MAGNA

Normal value <08 mm, borderline 08–10 mm and >10 mm abnormal.

SMALL BOWEL

Small bowel segments usually are less than 07 mm in diameter.

LARGE BOWEL

A large bowel segment which is more than 20 mm wide near term can be termed as abnormal.

PERICARDIAL FLUID

Minimal pericardial fluid is a normal finding after 20 weeks of gestation. So pericardial fluid of more than 02 mm is regarded as abnormal.

CUTANEOUS THICKNESS

Subcutaneous edema is diagnosed as abnormal when it measures more than 05 mm.

Measurement Methodology

AMNIOTIC FLUID INDEX ASSESSMENT

The uterus is divided into four quadrants by the midline and transverse axis and the amniotic fluid as the deepest vertical pocket free of fetal parts and umbilical cord is measured in each quadrant and all four quadrants add up to give the amniotic fluid index.

CHOROID PLEXUS

Choroid plexus occupies the whole of the body of the lateral ventricle. The anterior horn, body and posterior horn of the lateral ventricle should be measured. Measurement of any medial separation of the choroids plexus with the lateral ventricular wall should also be assessed for.

CEREBELLUM

The cerebellum is seen as a 'W' turned 90 degrees. The cerebellar hemispheres and the cerebellar vermis should be appreciated for posterior cranial fossa abnormalities. The cerebellar transverse diameter (CTD) is measured from the edges of both cerebellar hemispheres.

CISTERNA MAGNA

The cisterna magna is seen posterior to the cerebellar vermis and anterior to the occipital bone.

NUCHAL TRANSLUCENCY

The translucency (subcutaneous) between the skin and soft tissue posterior to the cervical spine has to be measured.

NUCHAL SKIN

The nuchal skin fold is measured from the posterior edge of the occipital bone and it includes the skin and the sonolucent area between the occipital bone and skin. Look in for any focal or diffuse thickening with/without septations.

CRANIAL BIOMETRY

Section for cranial biometry consists of the thalamus, the third ventricle and the cavum septum pellucidum.

- *Bi-parietal diameter:* Side to side measurement from the outer table of the proximal skull to the inner table of the distal skull.
- *Head perimeter:* The total cranial circumference, which includes the maximum antero-posterior diameter.
- *Occipito-frontal diameter:* Front to back measurement from the outer table on both sides.

ORBITAL MEASUREMENTS

- *Ocular diameter:* Measured from medial inner to medial lateral wall of the long orbit.
- *Interocular distance:* Measured from medial inner wall of one orbit to medial inner wall of the other orbit.
- *Binocular distance:* Measured from lateral inner wall of one orbit to lateral inner wall of the other orbit.

ABDOMINAL PERIMETER

In the section for abdominal perimeter measurement, the spine should be posterior and the umbilical part of the portal vein anterior.

Reporting

These are the parameters to be mentioned in the report. The list might appear too long but it is simple and one should routinely evaluate all these parameters.

Parameters to be routinely evaluated are mentioned as (R) and ones to be specifically looked in particular conditions are mentioned as (S).

FROM 05–10 WEEKS

- Uterine size (R)
- Location of gestational sac (R)
- Number of gestational sacs (R)
- Size of gestational sac (R)
- Yolk sac(R)
- Size of yolk sac (R)
- Embryo/fetus size (R)
- Menstrual age (R)
- Cardiac activity (R)
- Heart rate (R)
- Fetal movements (R)
- Trophoblastic reaction (R)
- Internal os width (R)
- Length of cervix (R)
- Any uterine mass (R)
- Any adnexal mass (R)
- Corpus luteum (present/absent) (R)
- Corpus luteum vascularity (S).

FROM 10–14 WEEKS

- Placental site (R)
- Liquor amnii (R)
- Fetal crown rump length (R)

- Menstrual age (R)
- Fetal movements and cardiac activity (R)
- Any gross anomalies (R)
- Nuchal translucency (R)
- Ductus venosus flow (S)
- Internal os width (R)
- Length of cervix (R)
- Any uterine mass (R)
- Any adnexal mass (R).

FROM 14–22 WEEKS

- Placenta (R)
- Liquor amnii (R)
- Umbilical cord (R)
- Cervix (R)
- Lower segment (R)
- Myometrium (R)
- Adnexa (R)
- Nuchal skin thickness (S)
- Cerebellar transverse diameter (S)
- Cisterna magna depth (S)
- Width of body of lateral ventricle (S)
- Inter-hemispheric distance (S)
- Ratio of the width of body of lateral ventricle to inter-hemispheric distance (S)
- Ocular diameter (S)
- Interocular distance (S)
- Binocular distance (S)
- Bi-parietal diameter (R)
- Occipitofrontal distance (R)
- Head perimeter (R)
- Abdominal perimeter (R)
- Femoral length (R)
- Humeral length (S)
- Foot length (S)
- Fetal movements and cardiac activity (R)
- Ductus venosus flow velocity waveform (S).

FROM 22–28 WEEKS

- All parameters of 14-22 weeks except nuchal skin fold thickness. (R) and (S)
- Umbilical artery and uterine artery flow velocity waveform. (S).

FROM 28–41 WEEKS

- Placenta (R)
- Liquor amnii (R)
- Umbilical cord (R)
- Cervix (R)
- Lower segment (R)
- Myometrium (R)
- Adnexa (R)
- Bi-parietal diameter (R)
- Occipitofrontal distance (R)
- Head perimeter (R)
- Abdominal perimeter (R)
- Femoral length (R)
- Distal femoral epiphysis (R)
- Biophysical profile (S)
- Color Doppler arterial (Umbilical artery, middle cerebral artery, descending aorta and both maternal uterine arteries) (S)
- Color Doppler venous (Umbilical vein, inferior vena cava and ductus venosus) (S).

Schematic Analysis for Fetal Anomalies

EXTRA-FETAL EVALUATION

Placenta	Umbilical cord	Liquor amnii
Thickness Location Morphology Focal masses	Number of vessels Origin and insertion Masses Length	Echo texture Quantity Amniotic bands
Cervix	Lower segment	Pelvis
Internal os Length serial evaluation	Thickness	Masses

FETAL EVALUATION

Choroid plexus	Cerebellum	Cisterna magna
Cysts Hydrocephalus Isolated dilatation	Cerebellar transverse diameter Superior and inferior cerebellar vermis Communication between fourth ventricle and cisterna magna	Depth Posterior fossa cyst
Orbits	Face	Nuchal skin
Hypo- and hypertelorism Lens	Lips Nostrils Ear	Thickness Septations
Spine	Heart	Thorax
Coronal Longitudinal Axial Ossification Soft Tissues	Situs Size Rate Rhythm Configuration Connections	Diaphragm Lung length Lung echoes Ribs Masses Cardiothoracic ratio

Contd...

Contd...

Abdomen	Skeleton	Biometry
Gastrointestinal	Cranium	Biparietal diameter
Hepatobiliary	Mandible	Occipito-frontal distance
Genitourinary	Clavicle	Head perimeter
Pancreas	Spine	Abdominal perimeter
Spleen	Extremities	Femoral length
		Humeral length

Fetal Abnormalities in Trisomy 21, 18 and 13

Organ system	Trisomy 21	Trisomy 18	Trisomy 13
Head and brain	Mild ventriculomegaly	Dolicocephaly Strawberry-shaped skull Large cisterna magna Choroid plexus cysts Agenesis of corpus callosum	Holoprosence-phaly Agenesis of corpus callosum Ventriculomegaly Enlarged cisterna magna Microcephaly
Facial	Flat face	Micrognathia Microphthalmia	Micrognathia Sloping forehead Cleft lip and/or palate Microphthalmia Hypotelorism
Neck	Thickened nuchal skin fold Cystic hygroma	Nuchal thickening	Nuchal thickening
Cardiac	Ventricular septa defect Atrial septal defects Atrioventricular canal Echogenic cardiac focus		Ventricular septa defect Atrial septal defect Dextrocardia Echogenic cardiac focus
Gastro-intestinal	Hyperechoic bowel Esophageal atresia Duodenal atresia Diaphragmatic hernia	Diaphragmatic hernia Omphalocele Esophageal atresia	Omphalocele

Contd...

Contd...

Organ system	Trisomy 21	Trisomy 18	Trisomy 13
Urogenital	Renal pyelectasis	Hydronephrosis, Horseshoe kidney	Renal cortical cysts Hydronephrosis Horseshoe kidney
Skeletal	Short femur and humerus Clinodactyly of fifth digit Widely spaced first and second toes Wide iliac angle	Clubfoot deformity Generalized arthrogryposis Clenched hands	Postaxial polydactyly Camptodactyly Overlapping digits
Hydrops/ cutaneous	Nonimmune hydrops		
Liquor amnii		Third trimester— polyhydramnios	Third trimester— hydramnios
Biometry		Second trimester— onset intrauterine growth retardation	Second trimester— onset intrauterine growth retardation
Doppler	Abnormal ductus venosus wave form	Abnormal ductus venosus waveform	Abnormal ductus venosus waveform

Appendix 6

Fetal Abnormalities in Triploidy and Turner's Syndrome

Organ system	Triploidy	XO
Head and brain	Ventriculomegaly Agenesis of the corpus callosum Dandy-Walker malformation Holoprosencephaly	
Spine	Meningomyelocele	
Facial	Hypertelorism Microphthalmia Micrognathia	
Neck	Cystic hygroma	Large, septate, cystic hygroma
Thorax		Pleural effusions
Cardiac	Septa! defects	Coarctation of the aorta
Gastrointestinal	Omphalocele	Ascites
Urogenital	Hydronephrosis	Horseshoe kidneys
Skeletal	Syndactyly of the third and fourth fingers Clubbed feet	Short femur Severe lymphoedema of all the soft tissues
Hydrops		
Placenta	Enlarged placenta or small, prematurely calcified placenta	
Liquor amnii	Oligohydramnios	
Biometry	Severe, early-onset, asymmetric intrauterine growth restriction (affecting the skeleton more than the head)	
Doppler	Abnormal umbilical artery Doppler waveform, showing a high-resistance pattern	

Fetal Abnormalities in Maternal Infections

Organ system	Cytomegalovirus	Rubella	Toxoplasmosis	Parvovirus
Head and brain	Ventriculomegaly Intracranial calcifications Microcephaly	Microcephaly	Ventriculomegaly Microcephaly Intracranial calcifications	
Facial		Cataracts Microphthalmia	Cataracts	
Cardiac	Cardiomegaly	Septal defects		Pericardial effusion
Gastrointestinal	Hyperechoic bowel Ascites Intrahepatic calcifications	Enlarged liver and spleen	Intrahepatic calcifications Hepatomegaly Ascites	Ascites
Hydrops	Hydrops			Hydrops
Placenta			Thickened placenta	Thickened placenta
Liquor amnii				Polyhydramnios
Biometry	Intrauterine growth restriction	Intrauterine growth restriction	Intrauterine growth restriction	

Table 1: Diagnosis of threatened abortion.

- Abdominal examination
  - Diffuse uterine tenderness
- Vaginal Examination
  - Vaginal bleeding which is usually mild
  - Closed cervical OS
  - Uterine size corresponds to period of gestation
  - No products of conception passed
  - No cervical movement pain
- Ultrasound examination
  - Intrauterine pregnancy with cardiac activity

Table 2: Diagnosis of inevitable abortion.

- Abdominal examination
  - Uterine tenderness
  - Contracting uterus
- Vaginal examination
  - Vaginal bleeding
  - Open cervical os and canal
  - Products of conception felt through cervical os
- Ultrasound examination
  - Products of conception entering or lying in the cervical canal.

Table 3: Diagnosis of incomplete abortion.

- History
  - Bleeding, pain, passage of tissue
- Abdominal examination
  - Uterine tenderness
- Vaginal examination
  - Uterine size smaller than expected
  - Open or closed internal os
  - Partial products of conception in process of being passed or lying in cervical canal
- Ultrasound appearance
  - Retained products of conception
  - Endometrium >5 mm thick
  - Echogenic or heterogeneous material
  - Vascularity present

Table 4: Diagnosis of complete abortion.

- History
  - Several hours of bleeding and pain and ease out of pain after passing tissue
- Abdominal examination
  - Mild uterine contractions
- Vaginal examination
  - Uterus small & contracted, cervix closed
- Ultrasound examination
  - Empty uterine cavity
- Examination of the abortions.

Table 5: Diagnosis of missed abortion.

- History
  - Symptoms of pregnancy may be absent or disappear
- Abdominal examination
  - Uterus may or may not be palpable, absent fetal heart sounds
- Vaginal examination
  - Uterus size is smaller than expected
  - Ultrasound examination
  - Empty sac
  - If fetus is present then
    Underdeveloped or small for date
    Absent cardiac activity

Table 6: Differences between various kinds of abortions.

Parameter	Threatened	Inevitable	Incomplete	Complete	Missed
• Bleeding	Mild	Heavy	Heavy	Heavy	Minimal (brownish)
• Abdominal pain	Mild	Moderate	Moderate	Moderate	Absent
• Uterine size gestational age	Corresponds	Corresponds	Size less than GA	Size less than GA	Size less than GA
• Cervical os	Closed	Open	Open	Closed/open	Closed
• Ultrasound	Live fetus	Products low in cavity	Small bits of products of conception felt	Cavity empty	Dead fetus/an/ anembryonic sac

Table 7: Ultrasound diagnosis of abortion.

In early pregnancy, a failed pregnancy can be suspected when certain sonographic criteria are not met using TVS. This is called "Discriminator level" and the absence of a finding at the discriminatory level predicts non-viable pregnancy.

Table 8: Discriminatory levels for early pregnancy.

Times of visualization	Expected finding on TVS
5 menstrual weeks	Gestation sac
5.5 menstrual weeks	Embryonic pole
Mean sac diameter 8–10 mm	Yolk sac
Crown rump length > 5 mm	Cardiac activity

Table 9: Ultrasound criteria for failed early pregnancy.

The diagnosis of failed early pregnancy can be based on following criteria:
- I. Gestation sac
  - No fetal pole or yolk sac in a gestational sac with mean sac diameter (MSD) > 25 mm
  - No change in MSD on consecutive scans 7 days apart
- II. Crown rump length (CRL)
Either of the following findings:
- No heart beat in an embryo with CRL ≥ 7 mm
- CRL < 7 mm and no interval growth over 5–7 days
- If there is doubt about fetal viability give the patient a benefit of doubt & USG repeated after 5–7 days.

Table 10: Ultrasound findings that may predict abortion.

Certain ultrasound findings are prediction of a failed pregnancy:
- Abnormal gestational sac
  - A gestational sac that is abnormally small or large
  - Irregular contour of gestational sac
  - Absence of double decidual sac sign
  - Low sac position in the uterus
- Abnormal yolk sac
  - A yolk sac large for gestational age
  - Irregular
  - Free floating in the gestational sac rather than at the periphery
  - Calcified
- Fetal bradycardia
  - Cardiac activity can be identified as early at ≥ 6 weeks of gestation @ 120–140 bpm
  - A FHR < 100 bpm at 6–7 weeks is bradycardia
  - Associated with 40% fetal loss
  - If FHR <70 bpm at 6–8 weeks, it predicts a 100% risk of fetal loss.
- Subchorionic hematoma
  - Collection of blood between the chorion & endometrium
  - Occur spontaneously or with bleeding P/V
  - Small hematomas does not increase risk of abortion but large ones.

  Large hematoma ≥ 25% of gestational sac increase risk of abortion, poor pregnancy outcomes, preterm premature rupture of membranes, preterm labor & stillbirth.

Table 11: Criteria used for ultrasonographic diagnosis of cervical insufficiency.

- Cervical length of < 25 mm between 16–24 weeks gestation
- Funnelling at the internal os
- Funnelling in response to the fundal pressure.

Table 12: Signs suggestive of ectopic pregnancy.

- General examination
  - Vital signs
  - Unruptured – stable or postural hypotension
  - Ruptured – Frank hypotension or hypovolemic shock
- Abdominal examination
  - Tenderness—diffuse/unilateral/bilateral
  - Peritoneal irritation from bleeding—abdominal guarding, rigidity, rebound tenderness, shifting dullness.
- Vaginal examination
  - Uterus – soft, slightly enlarged
  - Adnexal tenderness
  - Cervical movement pain
  - Bogginess in posterior fornix.
- Biochemical – serum hCG and discriminatory zone
  - If urine pregnancy test is positive but an intrauterine pregnancy is not demonstrated on TVS it is mandatory to get a serum hCG level
  - Commonly, with a serum hCG level of 1500–2000 mIU/mL a Ultra uterine pregnancy should be demonstrated by TVS. This is known as discriminatory zone of serum hCG level.
  - If serum hCG is lower than 1500 mIU/mL, the test is repeated in 48 hours. In a normal pregnancy hCG level will double in 48 hours, and an intrauterine pregnancy is demonstrable.
  - If hCG level does not double, repeat TVS to demonstrate a failing intrauterine pregnancy or an ectopic
- Transvaginal sonography
  - Gold standard for evaluation of ectopic
  - It can demonstrate an intrauterine pregnancy or an extrauterine pregnancy or may be nondiagnostic
  - Visualization of intrauterine pregnancy usually rules out ectopic except in case of heterotropic pregnancy
  - Extrauterine pregnancy is commonly seen as a mass lying between the ovary and the uterus.

USG findings suggestive of ectopic pregnancy in a Serum hCG positive (1500–200 mIU/mL)

Woman uterus

- Empty uterine cavity
- Pseudogestational sac/decidual cyst

Contd…

Contd...

- Adnexa
  - Simple adnexal cyst
  - Empty gestational sac (tubal ring)
  - Gestational sac with yolk sac and embryo
  - Cardiac activity 100% specific
  - Complex/solid adnexal cyst/mass
- Peritoneal cavity
  - Echogenic peritoneal fluid in the cul-de-sac
  - Doppler color flow mapping
  - "Ring of fire" sign: not specific
- Culdocentesis
  - It is the aspiration of the contents of the cul-de-sac to determine the presence of blood, done by a long 18 gauge needle passed through posterior fornix
  - Presence of non-clotting bloody fluid is suggestive of presence of bleeding ectopic pregnancy.
  - It is not usually performed now-a-days except where USG facility is not available or during emergency (woman in shock) for rapid diagnosis
- Diagnostic laparoscopy indications
  - If USG does not give specific diagnosis
  - If USG is unable to differentiate between an ectopic pregnancy and a bleeding ovarian cyst
  - Woman is hemodynamically unstable
  - If there is evidence of unruptured or ruptured ectopic pregnancy it can be tackled laparoscopically there and then
- Curettage
  - Presence of chorionic villi on curettage of the endometrium helps to diagnose an intrauterine pregnancy
  - It is however not used for diagnosis of ectopic pregnancy
- Serum progesterone
  - Serum progesterone level > 25 mg/mL suggests an intrauterine pregnancy
  - Level < 5 mg/ml indicates a nonviable intrauterine pregnancy or an ectopic pregnancy
  - Clinical usefulness of this test is doubtful.

Table 13: Diagnostic pathway for ectopic pregnancy.

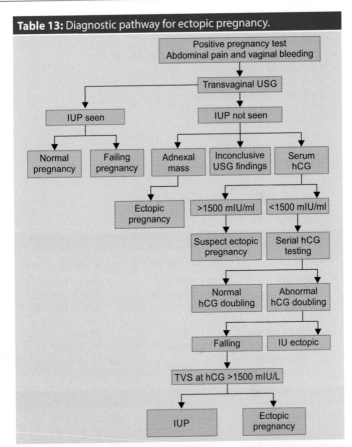

Table 14: Ultrasound features to confirm diagnosis of intra-uterine death.

- Absence of fetal cardiac activity
- Spalding's sign (collapse of fetal skill with overlapping bones)
- Hydrops
- Robert's sign (Intrafetal gas within the heart, great vessels, joints)
- Hyperflexion of the spine
- Crowding of the rib shadow
- Retroplacental dots in the presence of a massive abruption.

Table 15: Role of ultrasonography in twin pregnancy.

- Diagnosis of twins
- Determination of chorionicity and amnionicity
- Detection of fetal anomalies
- Evaluation of fetal growth
- Evaluation of fetal wellbeing
- Measurement of cervical length
- Guiding procedures
  - Selective termination
  - Selective feto reduction
  - Amniocentesis
  - Septostomy
  - Amnio reduction
  - Diagnosis of malpresentation
  - Assistance in labor

Table 16: Differences between monozygotic and dizygotic twins.

Parameter	Monozygotic	Dizygotic
• Phenotype	Identical	Non-identical
• Genotype	Identical	Non-identical
• Gender	Same	Same/different
• Incidence		
– Ethnic variation	Absent	Present
– Increase with ART	Minimal	Marked
– Adverse parental		
– Outcome	High	Low

Table 17: Determination of chorionicity

First trimester	Dichorionic	Monochorionic
• Gestational sac	Two	One
• Dividing membrane	Thick (> 2 mm)	Thin (< 2 mm)
Second trimester		
• Placenta	Two	One
• Fetal gender	Discordant	Concordant/discordant
Twin peak sign	Present	Absent
T sign	Absent	Present
Dividing membrane	Three or four layer	Two layers

Table 18: Sonographic criteria for diagnosis of twin to twin transfusion syndrome.

- Monochoriocity
- Same Gender
- Significant growth discordance
- Discrepancy in size of umbilical cord and amniotic fluid volume
- Cardiac dysfunction in recipient twin
    - Polyhydramnios (single deepest pocket >8 cm)
    - Oligohydromnios (single deepest pocket <2 cm)

Table 19: Quintero staging systems for TTTS.

- Stage I: Donor twin bladder visible
- Stage II: Donor twin bladder not visible, normal Doppler
- Stage III: Discordant amniotic fluid volumes, donor twin Bladder not visible, Abnormal Doppler studies of the umbilical artery, ductus venous or umbilical vein
- Stage IV: Ascites or trunk hydrops in either twin
- Stage V: Demise of either twin.

Table 20: Role of ultrasound in fetal growth restriction (FGR).

- Identification of FGR
    - By using growth charts
- Identification of type of FGR
    - Symmetric
    - Asymmetric
- Identification of cause
    - Infections
    - Structural abnormalities
    - Aneuploidy
- Antenatal surveillance
    - Amniotic fluid assessment
    - Biophysical profile
- Assessment of fetal size and 8 rate of growth
    - Using BPD, HC, AC and FL
    - Serial observation of biometric growth patterns (growth velocity)

Table 21: Further evaluation in FGR—role of ultrasound.

- Amniotic fluid volume
- Oligohydramnios is highly suggestive of FGR with increased risk of perinatal mortality
- Biophysical profile:
  - Helps in timing of delivery
- Uterine artery Doppler:
  - Reduced end diastolic flow
    » 30% of villus vasculature caused to function
    » Perinatal mortality still low
    » Safe to manage pregnancy expectantly
  - Absent/reversed flow
    » 60–70% Obliteration of placental arteries
    » Fetal hypoxia
    » Significant increase in perinatal morbidity and mortality
    » Should be delivered
- Middle cerebral artery Doppler
  - High diastolic flow (brain sparing effect) means fetal hypoxia
  - Ductus venosus Doppler
    » Absent or reversed ductus venosus (a wave) means impending acidemia and death.

Table 22: Classification of polyhydramnios.

- Mild
  - Vertical pockets of 8–11 cm
  - AFI of 25–30
- Moderate
  - Vertical Pockets of 12-15 cm
  - AFI of 30-35
- Severe
  - Vertical pockets of > 15 cm
  - AFI of > 35
  - Free floating fetus

Table 23: Evaluation of clinical polyhydramnios.

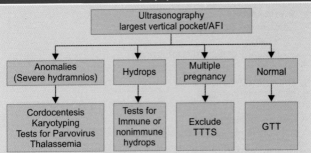

Ultrasonography largest vertical pocket/AFI

- Anomalies (Severe hydramnios) → Cordocentesis Karyotyping Tests for Parvovirus Thalassemia
- Hydrops → Tests for Immune or nonimmune hydrops
- Multiple pregnancy → Exclude TTTS
- Normal → GTT

Table 24: Evaluation of oligohydramnios.

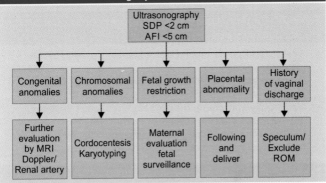

Ultrasonography SDP <2 cm AFI <5 cm

- Congenital anomalies → Further evaluation by MRI Doppler/ Renal artery
- Chromosomal anomalies → Cordocentesis Karyotyping
- Fetal growth restriction → Maternal evaluation fetal surveillance
- Placental abnormality → Following and deliver
- History of vaginal discharge → Speculum/ Exclude ROM

Table 25: Ultrasonographic signs of fetal anemia.

- Fetal MCA peak systolic velocity above 1.5 multiples of the median (MoMS)
- Polyhydramnios
- Hepatosplenomegaly
- Increased placental thickness
- Increased right atrial size
- Fetal hydrops (due to severe anemia & hydrops)
- Ascitis
- Pleural effusion
- Perichordial effusion
- Subcutaneous edema

Table 26: Features of hydrops fetalis.

- Severe anemia
- Congestive cardiac failure
  - Ascitis
  - Pleural & perichordial effusions
  - Subcutaneous & scalp edema
- Placental enlargement
- Hepatosplenomegaly
- Stillbirth
- Ultrasonography
  - Fluid in pleural, peritoneal and pericardial cavities
  - "Halo" around the neck due to scalp edema
  - Large placenta
  - Hepatosplenomegaly

Table 27: Current classification of placenta previa (on basis of ultrasonographic findings).

- *Total placenta previa:* Internal os is completely covered by the placenta
- *Partial placenta previa:* Internal os is partially covered by the placenta
- *Marginal placenta previa:* The placental edge comes up to the internal os but does not cover it.
- *Low lying placenta:* The placenta is in the lower segment but the placental edge is </= 2 cm from internal os.

Table 28: Ultrasonography in placenta previa.

- Transabdominal
  - Used for quick screening
  - Fundal placenta excludes placenta previa
  - 95% accuracy
  - False positive with a full bladder
  - False negative with fetal head low in the pelvis
- Transvaginal
  - Used for confirmation
  - 100% accuracy
  - Does not provoke bleeding
  - Tip of the transducer placed 2–3 cm below cervix
- Translabial
  - Alternative to transvaginal

Table 29: Sonographic findings of placenta accreta.

- Myometrial thickness (from serosa to retroperitoneal vessels) < 1 mm
- Large intraplacental blood lakes
- Loss of thinning of the normal hypoechoic area behind the placenta (clear space)
- Loss of normal continuous white line at serosal–bladder interface (bladder line)
- Focal modular projections into the bladder
- Color Doppler
  - Increase in vascular layer with turbulent flow
  - Hypervascularity of serosal bladder interface

Table 30: Significance of single umbilical artery (SUA).

- May Result from one of the following:
  - Primary Agenesis of one of the umbilical arteries
  - Secondary atresia or atrophy of a previously normal umbilical artery
  - Persistence of the original single allantonic artery of the body stalk
- Associated with anomalies
  - Genitourinary
  - Cardiac
  - Gastrointestinal
- When not associated with any anomalies – Good fetal outcome
- The outcome of SUA with associated anomalies or aneuploidy depends on the underlying chromosomal and structural abnormalities
  - Fetal karyotype should be offered when fetal anomalies are detected

Table 31: Ultrasound findings suggestive of fetal cytomegalovirus infection.

- Symmetric fetal growth restriction
- Cerebral ventriculomegaly
- Intracranial calcification
- Microcephaly
- Oligohydramnios/Polyhydramnios
- Hyperechogenic bowel
- Hepatic calcifications
- Hydrops fetalis/ascitis
- Pleural effusion
- Placental enlargement

Table 32: Indications for first trimester ultrasound.

- Location and documentation of pregnancy
- Assessment of gestational age by measuring
  - Gestational sac
  - Crown rump length
- Documenting cardiac activity
- Number of viable fetuses
  - Amniocity and chorionicity
- Identification of fetal anomalies
  - Acrania/anencephaly
  - Alobar holoprosencephaly
  - Major abdominal wall defects
- Uterine anatomy and adnexare
  - Uterine anomalies
  - Presence of fibroid
  - Ectopic Pregnancy
  - Adnexal masses
- Screening for aneuploidy (Chromosomal abnormality)
  - Nuchal translucency
  - Combined with biochemical screening.

Table 33: Gestational sac.

- Seen by TVS at 2–3 mm size
- Clearly visible at 4.5–5 weeks
- Gestational age (Days) = mean sac diameter (mm 0 + 30)
- Eccentric in location
- Surrounded by two rings of decidua

Table 34: Crown-Rump lengths.

- Most accurate for pregnancy dating
- Best measured between 7 and 10 weeks with an accuracy of ±3 days
- Can be measured between 11 and 14 weeks with an accuracy of ± 5 days

Table 35: Ultrasound imaging in twin pregnancy.

- 2 Placentas
    - Dizygotic twins
    - Dichorionic diamniotic
- Single placenta
    - Monozygotic twins
- Dichorionic twins
    - 2 sacs visible
    - Dividing membrane > 2 mm thick
- Monochorionic Diamniotic twins
    - Thin membrane
    - Difficult to see in first trimester
- Monochorionic Monoamniotic twins
    - Single amniotic cavity

Table 36: Measurement of Nuchal thickness (NT).

- Between 11 and 13th week
- Fetus in mid sagittal plane
- Fetal neck in neutral position
- Image magnified to feel screen with
    - Fetal neck
    - Head
    - Upper thorax

Table 37: Indications for second trimester ultrasound.

Transabdominal examination
- Fetus
    - Estimation of gestational age
    - Fetal biometry
    - Number/evaluation of multiple gestation
    - Screening for fetal anomalies
    - Evaluation of fetal growth

Amniotic fluid placenta
- Adjunct to prenatal diagnostic procedures
    - Amniocentesis
    - Chorionic villus sampling
    - Fetal blood sampling
    - Transvaginal USG
    - Evaluation of cervical insufficiency
    - Placental localization

Table 38: Correlation of accuracy of fetal age estimation with weeks of pregnancy.

Parameter used	Gestational age (weeks) at which the fetal age estimation is done	Accuracy of fetal age estimation (range in days)
Mean sac diameter	4.5–6	± 5–7
Crown rump length	7–10	± 3
BPD/HC/FL/AC	11–14	± 5
	14–20	± 7
	21–30	± 14
	> 30	± 21–28

Table 39: Components of a targeted/detailed fetal scan.

Head and Neck
- Midline falx and cavum septum pellucidum
- Lateral cerebral ventricles and choroid plexus
  - Ventriculomegaly
- Cerebellar hemispheres, vernices and cisterna magna
  - Banana sign
  - Dandy walker syndrome
- Nuchal fold thickness

Face
- Orbits
- Nose and nasal bone
- Mouth and lips

Spine
- Ossification centers
- Cervical widening
- Sacral tapering

Thorax
- Heart
- Four chamber view
- Outflow track
- Lungs
  - Intrathoracic masses or cysts
- Diaphragm
  - Diaphragmatic hernia

Contd...

Contd...

Abdomen
- Stomach (presence, size and sites)
- Liver
- Kidneys and bladder
- Bowel
- Umbilical cord insertion into fetal abdomen
- Umbilical cord vessel number
- Genitalia

Extremities
- Size, morphology and number.

Table 40: Indications for a third trimester ultrasound examination.

- Significant discrepancy between uterine size and clinical dates
  - Evaluation of fetal growth
- Assessment of fetal wellbeing
  - Amniotic fluid
  - Biophysical profile
  - Doppler evaluation
- Vaginal bleeding
  - Suspected placenta previa
  - Suspected placental abruption
- Multiple gestation
  - Suspected fetal death
  - Preterm rupture of membranes
  - Fetal wellbeing in an obese parturient
  - Estimation of fetal weights
  - Fetal presentation
  - Guidance to external cephalic version
  - Follow-up evaluation of fetal anomaly
  - Women registering late for antenatal care

Table 41: Indications for Doppler studies in obstetrics.

First Trimester
- Screening for aneuploidy
- As a marker for congenital heart disease
- Screening for pre-eclampsia

Second Trimester
- Screening for pre-eclampsia
- Identification of fetal anemia
- Evaluation of vascular malformations in the fetus and placenta
- Identification of cardiac and renal anomalies and diaphragmatic hernia

Third Trimester
- Evaluation of a growth restricted fetus
- Assessment of fetal hypoxia

Table 42: Scoring of biophysical profile.

	Normal (score = 2)	*Abnormal (score = 0)*
• Nonstress test	Reactive	Nonreactive
• Fetal breathing movements	• ≥ 1 episodes of rhythmic fetal breathing movements • Lasting ≥ 30 seconds • Within 30 minutes	No fetal breathing movements in 30 minutes
• Gross body movements	• ≥ 3 discrete body or limb movements • Within 30 minutes	< 3 movements in 30 minutes
• Fetal tone	• ≥ 1 episode of extension of fetal extremity with return to flexion OR Opening or closing of hand	No movements or slow movements
• Amniotic fluid volume	Single vertical pocket of amniotic fluid ≥ 2 cm	Largest single vertical pocket < 2 cm

Table 43: Interpretation and management of BPP score.

BPP score	Management
10/10	Low risk of developing fetal asphyxia
8/10 normal AFV	Low risk of developing fetal asphyxia
8/10 low AFV	• Consider chronic hypoxia • Repeat test or deliver
6/10	• Significant possibility of developing fetal asphyxia • If AFV abnormal—deliver • If AFV normal—repeat test and consider delivery
4/10	High risk of fetal asphyxia with one week—deliver
0–2/10	Certain fetal asphyxia—deliver

Table 44: Single deepest pocket measurement of amniotic fluid volume.

- Largest pocket
- Vertical measurement
- No cord or extremeties
- Part of biophysical profile

Table 45: Interpretation of single deepest pocket measurements.

- Oligohydramnios: Depth < 2 cm
- Normal: Depth ≥ 2 and < 8 cm
- Polyhydramnios: Depth ≥ 8 cm

Table 46: Interpretation of amniotic fluid/index.

- Oligohydramnios: AFI < 5 cm
- Normal: AFI >5 and < 24 cm
- Polyhydramnios: AFI ≥ 24 cm

Table 47: Rationale for modified biophysical profile.

- Less time consuming than BPP
- Measures 2 components
  - AFI which reflects chronic hypoxia
- NST which indicates acute hypoxia

Table 48: Interpretation of the modified biophysical profile.

- Normal
  - NST reactive
  - AFI, 5 or > 5 cm
- Abnormal
  - NST nonreactive
  - AFI < 5 cm

Table 49: Predictive value of Doppler velocimetry in ante partum fetal surveillance.

- Umbilical artery Doppler
  - Useful for fetal surveillance
  - Reduces the perinatal mortality in growth restricted fetus
  - No benefit in diabetes or post dated pregnancy
  - Used to decide on timing of delivery when BPP is abnormal or AFV is low
- Middle cerebral artery Doppler
  - Useful as an adjunct to umbilical artery Doppler
  - Brain sparing effect (Increased flow to brain)
  - Early sign of hypoxia
- Ductus venosus Doppler
  - Good but late predictor of poor perinatal outcome

Table 50: Sequential changes in fetal blood flow and biophysical of parameters in the presence of worsening hypoxia.

- Non reactive non stress test
  - Changes in doppler studies
    MCA: Brain sparing effect
    UA: Decreased/absent/reversed end diastolic flow
    DV: Abnormal flow
- Changes in BPP
  - Decreased fetal breathing movements
  - Decreased gross body movements
  - Decreased Fetal Tone

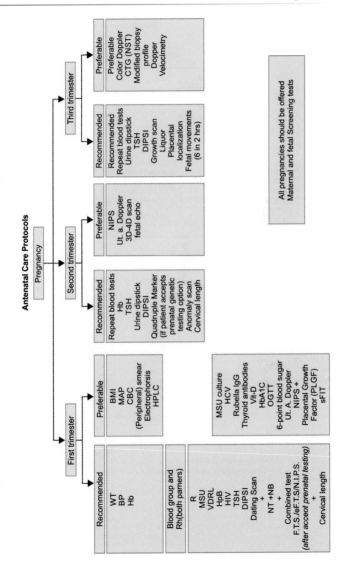

Antenatal Care Protocols

Pregnancy

First trimester

Recommended

WT
BP
Hb

Blood group and Rh(both partners)

R
MSU
VDRL
HpB
HIV
TSH
DIPSI
Dating Scan
+
NT +NB
+
Combined test
F.T.S./eF.T.S/N.I.P.S.
(after acceot prenatal testing)
+
Cervical length

Preferable

BMI
MAP
CBC
(Peripheral) smear
Electrophorsis
HPLC

MSU culture
HCV
Rubella IgG
Thyroid antibodies
Vit-D
HbA1C
OGTT
6-point blood sugar
Ut. A. Doppler
NIPS +
Placental Growth
Factor (PLGF)
sFIT

Second trimester

Recommended

Repeat blood tests
Hb
TSH
Urine dipstick
DIPSI
Quadruple Marker
(if patient accepts
prenatal genetic
testing option)
Anomaly scan
Cervical length

Preferable

NIPS
Ut. a. Doppler
3D-4D scan
fetal echo

Third trimester

Recommended

Repeat blood tests
Urine dipstick
TSH
DIPSI
Growth scan
Liquor
Placental
localization
Fetal movements
(6 in 2 hrs)

Preferable

Color Doppler
CTG (NST)
Modified biopsy
profile
Dopper
Velocimetry

All pregnancies should be offered
Maternal and fetal Screening tests

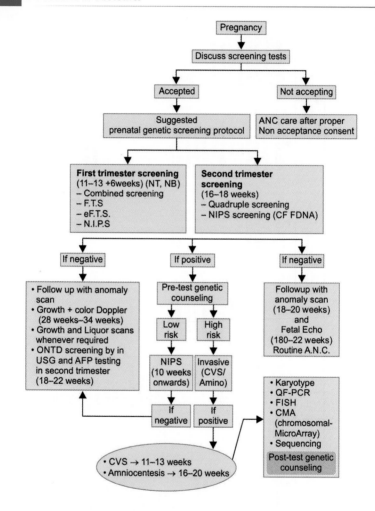

Index

Page numbers followed by *f* refer to figure and *t* refer to table